HEALING AMERICAN HEALTHCARE

LESSONS FROM THE PANDEMIC

WHERE DOES AMERICA GO FROM HERE?

John J. Dalton, FHFMA

Edward C. Eichhorn Jr.

September 20, 2021

This book is dedicated to the more than 3,600 frontline healthcare workers who have perished from Covid-19. They provided competent, compassionate care to those who had contracted it, often placing their own lives at risk given shortages of personal protective equipment and limited knowledge about Covid-19's transmissibility and lethality. To all of them – doctors, nurses, respiratory therapists, transporters, housekeepers, EMTs – we express our unending gratitude for their dedication. They truly are Healthcare Heroes!

I N MID-MARCH 2020 WHEN METRO NEW YORK JOINED MILAN AND MADRID AS THE EPICENTERS OF A GLOBAL pandemic, it became obvious to us that frontline healthcare workers would be facing enormous challenges for the foreseeable future. Time normally spent on professional development would be compressed to an unmanageable minimum. How could two retirees with a century of healthcare experience support them with timely information about important issues in a succinct manner?

We looked at the broad range of publications that deal with healthcare issues and realized that, even for retirees, the potential for information overload is endemic. The volume of new information published daily is overwhelming, whether it's professional journals (e.g., JAMA, New England Journal of Medicine, Lancet, etc.), studies and reports from credible sources (e.g., The Commonwealth Fund, Kaiser Family Foundation, Urban Institute, etc.) or media sources (NPR, Bloomberg, New York Times, Associated Press, Reuters, etc.). It's impossible to keep up.

Given our lifelong belief that access to affordable, quality healthcare is a fundamental human right and not just a privilege for those who can afford it, we launched the Healing American Healthcare Coalition and its twice monthly email newsletter, The Three Minute Read™, to provide subscribers with a "Reader's Digest" of five or six article summaries from major publications and other news sources.

Each day, we scan newsfeeds from several sources to select articles that might be of particular interest to busy healthcare professionals. The articles we've summarized fall into several distinct categories – the pandemic, whether global, in specific countries or the U.S., and provider, insurance and pharmaceutical issues. Some even touch on our favorite topic – universal healthcare. If an article summary piques a reader's interest, clicking on the title links to the full article in our e-book.

To date, we've published 41 issues summarizing 212 articles from more than 70 different sources. Looking back over the past 20 months by category, it was clear to us that the articles we had selected to summarize provide illuminating insights on various aspects of each topic. The book has nine chapters. The first eight cover specific topics with brief introductory comments followed by article summaries that portray the issue through the eyes of the journalists who reported on them. The U.S. response to the global pandemic is related in two chapters, separating the Trump administration response from the Biden administration response.

The final chapter discusses the lessons we have learned from the past 20 months. Whether our fellow Americans share these views has yet to be determined. Where do we go from here? In our opinion, building on the Affordable Care Act to provide access to affordable, quality healthcare for all Americans has never been more important. America remains the only member of the Organization for Economic Cooperation and Development (OECD) that does not do so. The Allcare Plan described in the first book in this series, "Healing American Healthcare: A Plan To Provide Quality Care To All While Saving $1 Trillion a Year," does so.

Thanks for your interest in the future of U.S. healthcare. The Covid-19 pandemic has put a fresh new light on many critical shortcomings that must be addressed to improve access to high quality care for all Americans. Please share with us any thoughts, concerns or suggestions that you have about the future of America's healthcare system at info@healingamericanhealthcare.org.

John Dalton & Ed Eichhorn
September 20, 2021

CONTENTS

CHAPTER 1

From Wuhan to the World – SARS-CoV-2 Goes Global

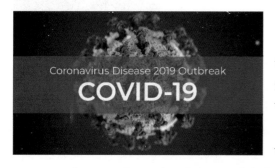

DECEMBER 31, 2019 – NEW YEAR'S EVE. AS REVELERS GATHERED IN New York's Times Square to welcome this century's "Roaring 20s," the World Health Organization's China Country Office was informed of cases of pneumonia of unknown cause detected in Wuhan City, Hubei Province of China.

Three weeks later, the United States confirmed its first case in Washington state – a man in his 30s developed symptoms after returning from Wuhan. Thus began a global roller coaster ride unlike any other since the Spanish flu pandemic of 1918-19 that originated in Kansas and took 675,000 American lives and roughly 50 million lives worldwide.

The World Health Organization (WHO) declared a global health emergency on January 30th and subsequently named the disease Covid-19, an acronym for coronavirus disease 2019. On March 11th, the WHO declared Covid-19 a global pandemic. Initial outbreaks in Milan and Madrid spread rapidly. During February, more than 2.2 million travelers arrived in New York from Europe, some already infected by the novel coronavirus. New Jersey's first case was confirmed March 5th. Shortly thereafter, the New York Metro Area joined Milan and Madrid as the global epicenters of the worst pandemic in over a century. By April, at least 82 countries had some form of lock-down in place according to UNICEF. On April 4th, the WHO reported that over 1 million cases of Covid-19 had been confirmed worldwide, a more than tenfold increase in less than a month.

Throughout the pandemic, the WHO periodically issued advice and guidance as the body of knowledge about SARS-CoV-2 grew rapidly. For example, on May 19th the WHO issued interim guidance on contact tracing. Similarly, on June 5th, the WHO published updated guidance on the use of masks for the control of Covid-19. With vaccine Emergency Use Authorizations very likely, on November 16th the WHO published interim guidance, developed with UNICEF, to help national governments in developing and updating their national deployment and vaccination plan for Covid-19 vaccines.

As 2021 began, the WHO's Strategic Advisory Group of Experts on Immunization (SAGE) met to review the vaccine data for the Pfizer/BioNTech vaccine and formulate policy recommendations on how best to use it. The vaccine was the first to receive an emergency use validation from WHO for efficacy against Covid-19.

The 31 articles summarized in this chapter cover a range of topics, including:

- the growing body of knowledge about the disease's unique symptoms (e.g., anosmia) and its treatment.
- role of governmental leadership in combating Covid-19.
- emergence of long-Covid.
- effectiveness of various mitigation measures.
- social media's spread of disinformation (e.g., it's just the flu); and
- factors contributing to the likeliness of an individual contracting Covid-19 (e.g., BMI>40, beware).

Sadly, by the end of August 2021, the origin of the deadly pathogen remained a mystery. Was it zoonotic disease transmission from a Wuhan "wildlife wet market" or an accidental leak from a lab? The Chinese government has been less than transparent in cooperating with global efforts to determine the source of SARS-CoV-2.

Fortunately, the WHO is setting up a Scientific Advisory Group for the Origins of Novel Pathogens, or SAGO to help establish frameworks for investigating the origins of pathogens early on as cases of disease are reported, as well as determining the origins of SARS-CoV-2.

Pandemic Global Three Minute Reads

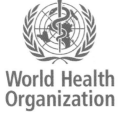

World Health Organization

WHO Sets 6 Conditions For Ending A Coronavirus Lockdown,
Bill Chapell, NPR 4/15/20

TMR Topline™ - With economic output stalled in many countries, pressure is building to ease lockdowns. According to UNICEF, at least 82 countries have some form of lockdown in place. WHO officials caution that, in many places, it's too soon to get back to normal. At a recent briefing, Dr. Mike Ryan, executive director of WHO's emergencies program said, *"You can't replace lockdown with nothing,"* stressed the importance of a committed and well-informed population and noted that we will have to change our behaviors for the foreseeable future. Any government that wants to start lifting restrictions must first meet six conditions:

1. Disease transmission is under control.
2. Health systems are able to "detect, test, isolate and treat every case and trace every contact."
3. Hot spot risks are minimized in vulnerable places, such as nursing homes.
4. Schools, workplaces and other essential places have established preventive measures.
5. The risk of importing new cases "can be managed."
6. Communities are fully educated, engaged and empowered to live under a new normal.

The WHO's goal is to taper restrictions so that governments can avoid a cycle of new Covid-19 outbreaks.

TMR's Take - The WHO's six conditions differ somewhat from the three phase "Opening Up America Again" guidelines announced by the Trump Administration last week. The guidelines are based on up-to-date data and readiness and are designed to mitigate the risk of resurgence and protect the most vulnerable.

Before proceeding to a phased reopening, states and regions must first show a decline of documented Covid-19 cases within a 14-day period and a robust testing program in place for at-risk health care workers. Throughout, individuals should continue to practice good hygiene with frequent hand washing, wearing face coverings in public, and staying home when sick.

For better, not worse, that is the new normal.

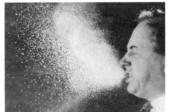

Identifying airborne transmission as the dominant route for the spread of COVID-19 by Renyi Zhang, Yixin Li, Annie L. Zhang, Yuan Wang and Mario J Molina. Proceedings of the National Academy of Sciences, June 11, 2020

TMR Topline™ - The authors studied the transmission pathways of the coronavirus by evaluating the trend and comparative mitigation efforts in the three first epicenters including Wuhan China, Italy and New York City. They found that that airborne transmission of the virus represents the most likely route to community spread of the disease. When considering the mitigation strategies of safe distancing, avoiding large gatherings and wearing a protective mask when in public, they found the most significant mitigation factor to reducing the spread of the virus was mandating face coverings. From 4/6 to 5/9 this practice reduced infections by 78,000 in Italy and by over 66,000 from 4/17 to 5/9 in New York City. Understanding the scientific basis for airborne transmission of this respiratory virus should dictate public policy to flatten the infection curve in the cities and states where hot spots are evolving.

The paper does not minimize the importance of all mitigation strategies to control the spread of Covid-19 including social distancing, avoiding crowds by staying at home and hand sanitizing are important. However, these measures were started in Italy and New York City well before mandating face coverings. Wuhan China implemented all these mitigation practices as well as extensive testing and contact tracing which lowered their infection curve more rapidly when compared with the other epicenters.

TMR's Take - The National Academy of Sciences study makes it clear that policy makers and political leaders throughout the U.S. need to be aware of and respect the science behind the community spread of Covid -19. Plans to reopen states and cities should heed the scientific findings on the importance of mitigation plans, especially wearing protective masks when in public areas.

What the Pandemic Reveals About the Male Ego by Nicholas Kristof, New York Times, 6/13/20

TMR Topline™ - The Pulitzer Prize winning columnist poses the question: *"Are female leaders better at fighting a pandemic?"* Kristof compiled data from 21 countries, 13 led by men and 8 led by women. The Covid-19 fatality rate was 214 per million in male-led countries and 36 per million in female-led countries including Denmark, Finland, Germany, Iceland, New Zealand, Norway and Taiwan. Noting that *"Virtually every country that has experienced coronavirus mortality at a rate of more than 150 per million inhabitants is male-led,"* Kristof attributes the difference to male *"ego and bluster"* and contrasts it with the low-key, inclusive and evidence-based leadership in countries led by women.

TMR's Take – The ancient adage *"Mother knows best"* appears to have merit. The fatality rate in male-led countries is six times higher! In previous issues, **TMR** summarized articles citing New Zealand's success in eliminating the virus and Germany's performance in controlling the pandemic.

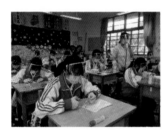

Some Countries Reopened Schools. What Did They Learn About Kids and Covid?, by Eric Miller, WIRED, 7/27/20

TMR Topline™ - The CDC has released school reopening guidelines that call for officials to reopen classrooms this fall, based on the idea that children do not become as sick from Covid-19 and are unlikely to transmit the virus to adults. Evidence from other countries that have reopened classrooms varies, suggesting that class size, distancing, the age of the students, and how prevalent the virus is locally are factors that must be considered. Neither Norway nor Denmark saw increased cases after reopening their schools in the late spring starting with younger students. Schools there boosted sanitizing procedures and limited class size, keeping children in small groups at recess and putting space between desks. Israel's experience was different – schools reopened with no masking or social distancing rules in place and class sizes up to 40 students. Since May, 125 schools have closed due to outbreaks.

A recent study of nearly 5,700 South Korean coronavirus patients found that children under 10 who were positive for Covid-19 had the lowest transmission rates of any age group, whereas children between 10 and 19 had transmission rates similar to adults. In Germany, physicians from Dresden University checked blood samples from 1,500 students and 500 teachers once schools reopened in May. Only 12 came back positive for antibodies to the coronavirus, indicating a low level of community infection. Even though coronavirus cases were detected in three of the 13 schools surveyed, the infection did not spread throughout the schools or the nearby community.

TMR's Take - The countries that have successfully reopened schools all have done a far better job of controlling the spread of Covid-19, with fatality rates a small fraction of the U.S.'s 46.2 per 100,000 at 7/30. Last week's report from the CDC about an outbreak at a sleepaway camp in Georgia is troubling. Of the 344 campers and staff for whom test results were available, 260 tested positive including over half ages 6-10, 44% ages 11-17 and one-third ages 18-21. The CDC report stated: *"The multiple measures adopted by the camp were not sufficient to prevent an outbreak. Relatively large cohorts sleeping in the same cabin and engaging in regular singing and cheering likely* *contributed to transmission. Use of cloth masks was not universal."* Teachers unions are expressing grave reservations about returning to classrooms this fall.

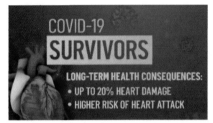

From 'brain fog' to heart damage, COVID-19's lingering problems alarm scientists, by Jennifer Couzin-Frankel, Science, 7/31/20

TMR Topline™ - Neuroscientist Athena Akrami, 38, has not been able to return to her London lab since contracting Covid-19 in March. Never hospitalized, her symptoms have waxed and waned; she struggles to think clearly and battles joint and muscle pain. SARS-CoV-2 uses a spike protein on its surface to latch onto cells' ACE2 receptors. The lungs, heart, gut, kidneys, blood vessels, and nervous system carry ACE2 on their cells' surfaces making them vulnerable to Covid-19. The virus can also induce a dramatic inflammatory reaction, including in the brain. The list of post-Covid problems include fatigue, a racing heartbeat, shortness of breath, achy joints, foggy thinking, a persistent loss of sense of smell, and damage to the heart, lungs, kidneys, and brain. Survivor studies are starting to probe them. Researchers in the U.K. will follow 10,000 survivors for one year to start, and up to 25 years.

Akrami collaborated with a group of Covid-19 survivors, to survey more than 600 who still had symptoms after 2 weeks, logging 62 different symptoms. A recent paper in JAMA Cardiology found that 78 of 100 survivors had cardiac abnormalities when their heart was imaged 10 weeks later. The article cites other survivor studies now underway in several countries.

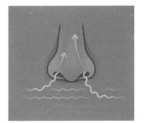

Going viral: What Covid-19-related loss of smell reveals about how the mind works, by Ann-Sophie Barwich, STAT, 8/14/20

TMR Topline™ - An olfactory specialist, Ms. Barwich criticizes the lengthy delay by the medical establishment in adding loss of smell (anosmia) to the official list of Covid-19 symptoms. At least half of confirmed cases worldwide had anosmia; in Germany, it was more than 2/3rds. An Iranian study found that 59 of 60 patients exhibited various smell dysfunctions.

TMR's Take - Infected by Covid-19? Your nose knows! Harvard professor of immunology Andrew Chan, co-founder of the Covid Symptom Study, concludes that the strongest predictor of a Covid-19 infection is a loss of taste or smell, a symptom that is relatively uncommon in other viral syndromes. Decreased smell function is a major marker for the SARS-CoV-2 infection. Smell testing should be used for early identification of Covid-19 patients in need of early treatment or quarantine.

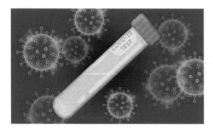

Clues to Why COVID-19 Hits Men Harder Than Women by Robert Preidt, 8/28/20 HealthDay News

TMR Topline™ - Covid-19 infects men at a higher rate and men have more difficult outcomes than women. Dr. Akiko Iwasaki, Professor of Immunology and Molecular Biology at the Howard Hughes Medical school at Yale University, led a research team that examined how men and women's immune systems respond to this virus infection.

In evaluating nasal, saliva and blood samples from both Covid-19 patients and healthy individuals, the researchers found that men develop higher cytokine levels and women generally develop higher T-cell levels as an early response. The cytokine reaction can cause an inflammation that attacks the virus in the lungs but also results in reduced oxygen levels and fluid buildup that can cause other organs to fail. T-cells are white blood cells that attach to viruses. Older men do not develop T-cell responses as well as younger people. Older women can also develop higher cytokine reactions and therefore can have worse outcomes than other women who do not.

Dr. Iwasaki has said these findings *"suggest we need different strategies to ensure that treatments and vaccines are equally effective for both men and women."* For example, when a vaccine has been approved, younger women may develop immunity from just one vaccine injection while older men might require as many as three injections to develop immunity. Dr. Amesh Adalja, an infectious disease expert at Johns Hopkins University commented, *"We are increasingly seeing that a one-size-fits-all strategy is not always possible, and precision medicine -- based on each individual's unique characteristics -- is likely the best approach."*

TMR's Take –The Yale findings in this study clearly point out that the basic understanding of how the immune system responds to this virus based on both sex and age is crucial to learning how care givers can produce better outcomes in treating Covid–19.

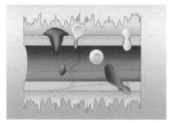

A Supercomputer Analyzed Covid-19 — and an Interesting New Theory Has Emerged, by Thomas Smith, Elemental, 9/1/20

TMR Topline™ - Oak Ridge National Labs opened in 1943 as the research site for the Manhattan Project that developed the atomic bomb. Today, it has provided what scientists are describing as a "eureka moment" in identifying how Covid-19 impacts the body. Site of the world's second fastest supercomputer, scientists crunched data on more than 40,000 genes from 17,000 genetic samples analyzing 2.5 billion genetic combinations. It took more than a week, leading to the bradykinin hypothesis that provides a model that explains many of Covid-19's bizarre symptoms.

It also suggests more than ten potential treatments, including some that are FDA approved. Generally, a Covid-19 infection begins when the virus enters the body through ACE2 receptors in the nose, then proceeds through the body entering cells where ACE2 also is present. Its insidious progression is well documented in this fascinating article.

TMR's Take - The research team's finding may well be the 21st century equivalent of the Manhattan Project. The bradykinin hypothesis provides a unified theory for how Covid-19 works. Dr. Daniel Jacobson, lead researcher is clear: "*We have to get this message out.*" **TMR** agrees.

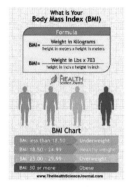

Doctors studying why obesity may be tied to serious COVID-19, by Candice Choi, Associated Press, 9/8/20

TMR Topline™ - There's some evidence that obesity itself can increase the likelihood of serious complications from a coronavirus infection. One study of more than 5,200 infected people, including 35% who were obese, found that the chances of hospitalization rose for people with higher BMIs, even when considering other conditions that could put them at risk. The increased risk for serious Covid-19 illness appears more pronounced with extreme obesity, or a BMI of 40 or higher. Multiple factors make it more difficult for obese individuals to fight the coronavirus, including chronic inflammation and how fat is distributed in the body.

TMR's Take - BMI>40? Beware of Covid-19!.

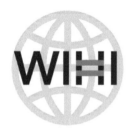

Measuring the COVID-19 Policy Response Around the World, by Avik Roy, Foundation for Research on Equal Opportunity

TMR Topline™ - The Foundation for Research on Equal Opportunity conducted an in-depth review of per capita fatality rates in 31 high income countries. Variables considered included stringency of economic restrictions, relative isolation and type of universal healthcare. It found no correlation between the format of a country's health insurance system and its ranking. Among countries with single payer systems, Australia fared well, but Italy, Spain and the U.K. did not. Countries with private insurance and/or consumer-driven models are also all over the rankings.

Overall, five Pacific Rim countries (Hong Kong, Korea, Japan, Singapore, Taiwan, and New Zealand) nations fared the best in the review's Pandemic Performance rankings. Except for Germany, the major Western democracies (France, Italy, Spain, the U.K. and the U.S.) did not. A key factor in successfully controlling Covid-19 was SARS "muscle memory." Residents of the five countries were acutely aware of the threat posed by Covid-19 due to their prior experience with the SARS-CoV pandemic in 2002-03. Asian governments took the threat more seriously early on, and enacted aggressive contact tracing measures and had already built up stockpiles of personal protective equipment.

TMR's Take - The Foundation also compiles a FREOPP World Index of Healthcare Innovation. The U.S. is ranked #4 behind Switzerland, Germany, and the Netherlands—three countries with universal private health insurance. Different criteria – different results!

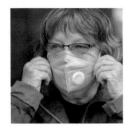

Facial Masking for Covid-19 — Potential for "Variolation" as We Await a Vaccine, by Monica Gandhi, M.D., M.P.H. and George W. Rutherford, M.D., New England Journal of Medicine, 9/8/20

TMR Topline™ - The authors hypothesize that in addition to reducing the probability of infection, universal face masking may also reduce the severity of SARS-CoV-2 among people who do become infected by making a greater proportion of them asymptomatic. They cite a long-standing theory of viral pathogenesis, which holds that the severity of disease is proportionate to the viral inoculum received. Wearing masks could be a form of "variolation" that slows the spread of the virus by reducing the viral inoculum to which the wearer is exposed and the subsequent clinical impact of the disease. Variolation was a 19th century process of trying to protect patients from smallpox by infecting them with a small amount of the virus before the development of vaccines.

TMR's Take - Earlier studies published by the National Academy of Sciences and Health Affairs (see TMR, June 2020-2) documented airborne transmission as the most dominant route for the spread of Covid-19. This theory reinforces the overall importance of universal mask wearing in public places. While multiple studies confirm the effectiveness of wearing face masks in public as a mitigation measure, only 45% of Americans wear masks on a regular basis.

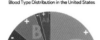

More Evidence Points to Role of Blood Type in COVID-19, by Molly Walker, Associate Editor, MedPage Today October 14, 2020

TMR Topline™ - Two recent studies shed additional light on the role that blood type may play in Covid-19. A Danish study found that blood type O was associated with reduced risk of developing Covid-19. Writing in *Blood Advances,* the authors found no increased risk for hospitalization or death associated with blood type. However, a smaller study from six metropolitan Vancouver hospitals from February 21st to April 28th found that blood types A or AB were associated with increased risk for mechanical ventilation, continuous renal replacement therapy, and prolonged ICU admission than patients with blood type O or B. Inflammatory cytokines did not differ between groups. Both groups acknowledged prior research findings that certain blood groups were linked to virus susceptibility and that more extensive studies are needed to infer causality.

TMR's Take - Further research is needed on the role of blood types in the risk for contracting and the severity of the course of a Covid-19 infection.

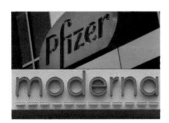

Moderna, Pfizer Shots Look Strong. Here's How They Stack Up, by James Paton, Bloomberg 11/16/20

TMR Topline™ -The encouraging late-stage trial results from Pfizer and Moderna have set a high bar for rival vaccines soon to follow.

How do the results compare? Moderna's vaccine was 94.5% effective in a preliminary analysis, slightly higher than the 90% reported earlier by Pfizer and its partner, BioNTech SE. Both use messenger RNA technology that instructs cells to make copies of the coronavirus spike protein stimulating the creation of protective antibodies.

What are the storage and distribution challenges? Pfizer's vaccine requires deep freeze storage but can be kept at refrigerator temperatures for as much as five days. Moderna's vaccine is stable at refrigerator temperatures for 30 days.

When could they be ready to deploy? Both companies are expected to seek emergency-use authorization from the U.S. Food and Drug Administration.

What are the big questions that remain? It's unclear how long protection will last or how many will refuse to be vaccinated. Ramping up production and distributing the doses also pose challenges.

TMR's Take - On 11/23, Astra-Zeneca announced that its vaccine developed in the U.K. with Oxford University can protect 70.4% of people from becoming ill and up to 90% if a lower first dose is used. The development of three promising vaccines in so short a period of time is an incredible achievement. Production and distribution challenges remain, but this is an important first step.

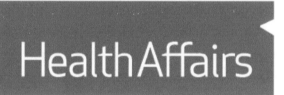

Clinical Outcomes Of A COVID-19 Vaccine: Implementation Over Efficacy, by A. David Paltiel, Jason L. Schwartz, Amy Zheng and Rochelle P. Walensky, Health Affairs 11/19/20

TMR Topline™ - Researchers from Yale and Harvard. examined vaccine efficacy, with variables of implementation effectiveness and background epidemic severity. They reviewed how these potential outcomes could impact total infections, hospitalizations, and deaths. Using mathematical simulations, they found that factors related to implementation will contribute more to the success of vaccination programs than a vaccine's efficacy as determined in clinical trials. They learned that the benefits of a vaccine will decline if manufacturing or deployment delays, significant concerns in the public about getting vaccinated or greater epidemic severity develops. They found that there is an urgent need for health officials to continue and expand efforts to promote public confidence in Covid-19 vaccines, and to encourage continued adherence to other mitigation approaches, even after a vaccine becomes available.

When interviewed by *The New York Times* about the study, Dr. Paltiel said *"Vaccines don't save lives. Vaccination programs save lives."* His study team concluded that to reduce the pandemic's infections, hospitalizations and deaths, a successful vaccine rollout was just as important as the vaccine's efficacy. Dr. Paltiel is concerned that the U.S. has not done enough to prepare for successful distribution of the vaccine in the months to come after one or more vaccines are approved for use.

TMR's Take - This study makes it clear that mitigation recommendations (wear masks in public, avoid crowds, wash hands frequently) along with a successful rollout of approved vaccines and public commitment to getting vaccinated are all important to controlling Covid-19.

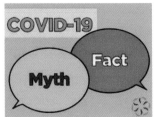

8 facts about the coronavirus and COVID-19 to counter misinformation, by Marisa Iati, *The Washington Post*, 12/6/20

TMR Topline™ - Social media spreads misinformation about COVID-19. The writer documents 8 key facts:

Masks help prevent the spread of coronavirus. Several studies support the theory that face coverings reduce the risk of infection. In Senate testimony in September, CDC Director Dr. Redfield said that masks are "*the most important, powerful public health tool we have*" for combating the pandemic.

There are no known cures for Covid-19. Many false rumors have circulated about potential cures, ranging from drinking bleach to snorting cocaine. The FDA has issued nearly 150 warning letters to companies making fraudulent misrepresentations.

Hospitals have no reason to purposely diagnose Covid-19 inaccurately. Rumors persist that hospitals are gaming the system to obtain higher payments. The CARES Act did include a provision to reimburse hospitals more for uninsured coronavirus patients and those with Medicare. The reality is that hospitals are probably losing money on Covid-19 patients because the illness is difficult to treat and many hospitals have been overwhelmed by a surge of people needing care.

The coronavirus is more deadly than influenza. About 2 percent of diagnosed coronavirus cases are lethal, but only 0.1 percent of seasonal flu cases are lethal.

The coronavirus vaccine candidates do not affect people's DNA. Both the Pfizer/BioNTech and Moderna vaccines are based on genetic material called messenger RNA. That mRNA teaches the body's cells to build protein on the surface of the coronavirus, therefore making the immune system recognize and block the true virus. According to the CDC, vaccines using mRNA do not "affect or interact with" a person's DNA.

Staying home, using hand sanitizer, and washing our hands more often are healthy. The assertion that limiting time with people outside our households could damage our ability to fight diseases may stem from the "hygiene hypothesis." Scientists at the Cleveland Clinic say there is no evidence that temporarily increasing these hygiene routines is damaging.

Scientists believe the coronavirus originated in animals. Scientific evidence strongly supports the conclusion that the virus was not man-made in a Chinese laboratory; its genome suggests that it is naturally occurring in nature. The CDC, WHO and DNI investigations also support this conclusion.

Urging high-risk people to stay home and letting everyone else live normal lives would not "solve" the crisis. Letting people interact freely, as if there were no pandemic, would enable the virus to travel through the population even more quickly, straining the capacities of already overwhelmed hospitals and burned-out health-care workers. About 21% of adults over 65 live in multigenerational households – isolating the vulnerable simply is not practical.

TMR's Take - It's no surprise that the fact-checking site Politifact named "*Coronavirus Downplay and Denial*" as its Lie of the Year. It's well worth reading.

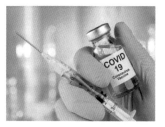

Once you and your friends are vaccinated, can you quit social distancing?, by Sigal Samuel, VOX, 1/12/21

TMR Topline™ - If you think that eliminating the Covid-19 pandemic is as a simple as get the shot then get rid of the virus, Eleanor Murray, a Boston University epidemiologist disagrees: *"Realistically, it's definitely not going to be an on/off switch on normal."* The best way to set realistic expectations around what life will look like in 2021 is to think of it in three stages. Stage 1 is what you can safely do once you and your close friends and family are vaccinated. Stage 2 is what you can safely do once your city or state has reached herd immunity, Stage 3 is what you can do once herd immunity is reached internationally.

Stage 1: You and your close friends or family are vaccinated. Can you all rent a cabin in the woods and spend a weekend together, without masks or social distancing? Realistically, not until at least a week after all have received the second shot. The risk would be relatively low, provided no one has underlying conditions and doesn't live with vulnerable unvaccinated people who need to be protected from infection. But no barhopping!

Stage 2: Your city or state has reached herd immunity. Dr. Fauci says that Americans should continue with masking and social distancing until 75 to 85 percent of the population is vaccinated, which is not likely to happen until mid-Fall. It's likely that regions within the U.S. will pass the immunity threshold at different times, so mask wearing will need to continue. When it comes to the coronavirus, nobody is truly safe until everybody is safe.

Stage 3: Herd immunity is reached internationally, not likely to be reached until 2022 or later given the unequal access to vaccines around the world. According to Dr. Murray, *"It's really going to come down to what we learn over the next few months about how well the vaccine prevents infection and transmission."*

TMR's Take –Reaching herd immunity will not happen all at once; that African safari you may have been planning will have to wait a while. However, if Americans step up and get vaccinated, 2021's Thanksgiving and Christmas holidays are likely to be much closer to normal.

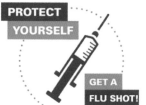

Impact of the Influenza Vaccine on COVID-19 Infection Rates and Severity, by Anna Conlon, PhD, Carmel Ashur, MD, MS, Laraine Washer, MD, Kim A. Eagle, MD, Marion A. Hofmann Bowman, MD, American Journal of Infection Control, 2/22/21

TMR Topline™ - The study found that people who received the influenza vaccine were less likely to test positive for Covid-19, and if they were infected with the virus, they were less likely to need hospitalization, mechanical ventilation, or a longer hospital stay. The researchers studied a retrospective cohort of 27,201 patients who were tested for Covid-19 from 2/27-7/15/20 in the Michigan Medicine healthcare system. The research suggests a possible association between the influenza vaccine and decreased risk of Covid-19 with improved clinical outcomes.

TMR's Take - Whether it was the prevalence of masking and social distancing, or a high level of flu vaccinations, America has avoided the dreaded *"twindemic."* As of early February, only 1,363 confirmed cases were reported compared with an average of 401,000 at the same time during the five prior flu seasons.

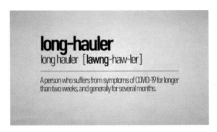

Do Vaccines Help COVID Long-Haulers?, by Kristina Fiore, MedPage Today 3/4/21

TMR Topline™ - Some people suffering from long Covid have found significant symptom relief after their first dose of the Covid-19 vaccine. New York Times Editorial Board member Mara Gay is one, feeling significantly better after her first vaccine dose. Hannah Davis, co-chief of Patient-Led Research for Covid-19, said her organization is currently working on a survey to study the phenomenon. In a U.K. survey, 16% of patients said their long Covid symptoms had improved by 2 weeks after their first dose.

Akiko Iwasaki, PhD, of Yale University believes that a study is worth considering, given that it could potentially confirm vaccination as a therapy for long Covid. Last June, Iwasaki proposed three potential mechanisms for long Covid: a persistent viral reservoir; viral fragments or remnants that drive inflammation; or an autoimmune response induced by the infection. Stanley Weiss, MD, an infectious disease specialist and epidemiologist at Rutgers New Jersey Medical School, agrees: *"The way you progress in science and medicine, is that you take observations from astute observers and pursue them with scientific rigor."*

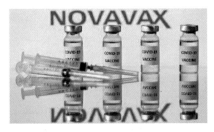

Novavax vaccine 96% effective against original coronavirus, 86% vs British variant in UK trial, by Dania Nadeem, Carl O'Donnell, Reuters, 3/11/21

TMR Topline™ - A late-stage trial in the U.K. found Novavax's vaccine 96% effective against Covid-19's original variant and 86% effective in protecting against the more contagious B.1.1.7 variant. In South Africa, it was 55% effective, but still fully prevented severe illness. The U.K. trial enrolled more than 15,000 people aged 18 to 84, assessing the vaccine's efficacy during a period with high transmission of the U.K. virus variant now circulating widely. Novavax expects data from a 30,000-person trial in the United States and Mexico by early April. The vaccine could be cleared for use in the United States as soon as May if U.S. regulators decide the U.K. data is enough to make a decision.

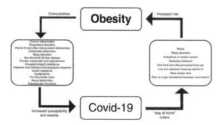

Most virus deaths recorded in nations with high obesity levels: analysis, by Joseph Choi, the Hill, 03/04/21

TMR Topline™ - The World Obesity Federation's annual report found a connection between increased Covid-19 deaths and high obesity rates. *"Comparing countries around the globe we find a close association between deaths from Covid-19 and the prevalence of overweight in the adult population,"* the WOF said in its analysis of the research. The WOF is associated with the World Health Organization and found that the connection between increased risk of severe Covid-19 cases or death and higher bodyweight was observed across multiple countries. A U.S. study reported that obese people were twice as likely to be hospitalized with Covid-19 and six times more likely to die after developing the disease. The organization ruled out potential explanations for the correlation between obesity and severe Covid-19 cases such as old age, wealth and increased reporting, saying the link appeared to be independent of these factors.

TMR's Take - A Brookings Institution study looked at the difference between advanced and developing economies last year, concluding: *"a large part of the positive correlation between income and deaths per million is due to …the age distribution and obesity."* Put simply, America's obesity epidemic will continue to plague the U.S. as the primary public health challenge post-pandemic.

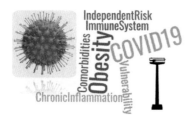

Stay-at-Home Orders Linked to Weight Gain, by Jeff Minerd, Contributing Writer, MedPage Today, 3/22/21

TMR Topline™ - A study led by Gregory Marcus, MD at University of California San Francisco found that Americans gained weight at a rate of about 1.5 pounds/ month after being told to stay out of public places. Published in JAMA Network Open, the authors noted: *"It is important to recognize the unintended health consequences SIP [shelter-in-place] can have on a population level."* Study participants resided in 37 U.S. states and DC. Marcus said the weight gain problem may persist even after SIP restrictions have been lifted.

TMR's Take - Those who have sent children off to college are all too familiar with the *"freshman 15"* pounds, but the *"Covid 19"* is far more concerning given that 36.2% of American adults were obese pre-pandemic. **TMR's** previous issue noted the connection between increased risk of severe Covid-19 cases or death and higher bodyweight, citing a study that found that obese people were twice as likely to be hospitalized with Covid-19 and six times more likely to die after developing the disease.

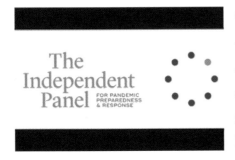

COVID-19 Was 'A Preventable Disaster,' WHO-Ordered Report Says, by Bill Chappell, NPR, 5/12/21

TMR Topline™ - An independent review ordered by the World Health Organization found that the Covid-19 pandemic exposed dangerous failings on both the national and international scale. The Independent Panel for Pandemic Preparedness and Response said Covid-19 was *"a preventable disaster."* It said the WHO lacks the power to investigate and act swiftly when confronted with potential outbreaks, calling February 2020 *"a lost month"* when countries could have acted to contain the coronavirus and prevent the pandemic's worst effects. The panel's recommendations included asking high-income countries to provide at least 1 billion vaccine doses to middle-income countries and more than 2 billion doses by the middle of 2022. It also urged formation of a Global Health Threats Council and a system for outbreak surveillance that is based on full transparency.

TMR's Take: The *"preventable disaster"* leaves American healthcare facing a perfect storm as it recovers: a critical need to expand primary care when women are leaving healthcare and telehealth may increase nurses' workloads. Dr. Yalda Jabbarpour, a primary care doctor who studies family medicine policy said *"It's really important that our healthcare system revamps and thinks about what women in the workforce need. The pandemic has brought that to light."* **TMR** agrees.

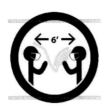

Experts say those who are not inoculated against Covid-19 shouldn't rely on protection from those who are, by Madeline Holcombe, CNN, 5/25/21

TMR Topline™ - As the U.S. reaches major Covid-19 vaccination milestones, health experts warn that unvaccinated individuals should not rely on protection from those who have been inoculated, as their infection risk remains the same as during the January surge. *"The work ahead of us is going to be really challenging, we still have to keep on convincing individuals who are not yet vaccinated that they are not safe,"* CNN medical analyst Leana Wen said. *"The pandemic is not over for them."*

According to the CDC, half of the U.S. adult population is fully vaccinated. For them, the upcoming Memorial Day weekend may be like it was before the pandemic. CDC Director Dr. Rochelle Walensky said, *"We are on a good downward path, but we are not quite out of the woods yet."* Dr. Wen advised that unvaccinated people keep masking, social distancing and practicing precautions.

TMR's Take - Sadly, the unvaccinated continue to be at risk of contracting Covid-19 and stressing an already overburdened healthcare system.

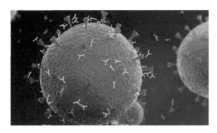

Immunity to the Coronavirus May Persist for Years, Scientists Find, by Apoorva Mandavilli, New York Times, 5/26/21

TMR Topline™ - Two recent studies report that immunity to the coronavirus lasts at least a year and possibly a lifetime, improving over time especially after vaccination. These findings may reduce fears that protection against the virus could be short-lived. Indications are that most people who have recovered from Covid-19 and who later were immunized will not need boosters. Those who were vaccinated but never infected likely will need booster shots. A small number of those infected who did not have a large immune response may also need booster shots.

Cells that retain a memory of the virus are in the bone marrow and may produce antibodies in response to an infection of the virus at any time according to the study published on Monday in the journal Nature. The second study, posted online at BioRxiv, found that memory B cells continue to mature and strengthen for at least one year after the infection. *"The papers are consistent with the growing body of literature that suggests that immunity elicited by infection and vaccination for SARS-CoV-2 appears to be long-lived,"* said Scott Hensley, an immunologist at the University of Pennsylvania who was not a part of these research projects. Dr. Michel Nussenzweig, an immunologist at Rockefeller University in New York who led the study on memory maturation said, *"People who were infected and get vaccinated really have a terrific response, a terrific set of antibodies,"* He also said, *"I expect that they will last for a long time."*

TMR Take – Fully vaccinated Americans can breathe a sigh of relief - they have little to fear from breakthrough infections. It's likely that booster shots may be needed in future years, like the seasonal flu shots. Recovered Covid patients may not need them.

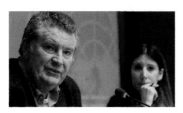

WHO says delta is the fastest and fittest Covid variant and will 'pick off' most vulnerable, by Berkeley Lovelace, Jr., CNBC, 6/22/21

TMR Topline™ - First identified in India, the Delta variant of the coronavirus has spread to 92 countries, replacing the highly contagious Alpha variant that swept across Europe and later the U.S. earlier this year. According to Dr. Michael Ryan, executive director of the WHO's health emergencies program, *"This particular delta variant is faster, it is fitter, it will pick off the more vulnerable more efficiently than previous variants."* Ryan said world leaders and public health officials can help defend the most vulnerable through the donation and distribution of Covid vaccines. He described the fact that we haven't as *"a catastrophic moral failure at a global level."* The Biden administration is donating 55 million vaccine doses. Most will be distributed through COVAX, the WHO-backed immunization program.

TMR's Take - Heed the doctors lifesaving advice! If you haven't already done so, ***get vaccinated!*** The life you save may be your own

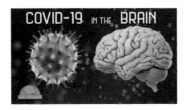

New Covid study hints at long-term loss of brain tissue, Dr. Scott Gottlieb warns, by Emily DiCiccio, CNBC, 6/17/21

TMR Topline™ - Citing a new study from the U.K., former FDA Director Dr. Scott Gottlieb warned about the potential for long-term brain loss from post-Covid, stating, *"the study suggests that there could be some long-term loss of brain tissue from Covid, and that would have some long-term consequences."* The U.K. study examined brain imaging before and after a coronavirus infection and looked specifically at the potential effect on the nervous system. Gottlieb said that the destruction of brain tissue could explain why Covid patients lost their sense of smell.

TMR's Take - For nearly one of four Covid survivors, beating the infection is not the end of the battle. For some, the symptoms continue to persist and may last for years. Preventing the next pandemic should be the #1 priority on any public health agenda.

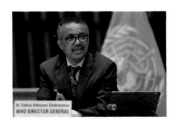

WHO calls for a temporary moratorium on administering booster shots of Covid-19 vaccines, by Helen Branswell, STAT, 8/4/21

TMR Topline™ - The World Health Organization called for a two-month moratorium on the use of Covid-19 vaccine booster shots by wealthy countries. Director-General Tedros Adhanom Ghebreyesus said that the delay would get enough vaccine supply into COVAX, the WHO-led international distribution system, to vaccinate 10% of all countries populations, especially those at highest risk. More than 80% of the 4 billion vaccinations to date have been in high income countries. Currently it is not clear that booster doses are needed.

TMR Take –Why not provide booster shots to the 7 million immunocompromised Americans ***and*** honor the WHO's moratorium request? While Moderna and Pfizer both are urging booster shots after 6 months, data shows their vaccines retain a high degree of effectiveness. By September month-end more data will be available to decide whether booster shots are needed.

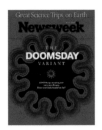

A Doomsday COVID Variant Worse Than Delta and Lambda May Be Coming, Scientists Say, by David H. Freeman, Newsweek, 8/4/21

TMR Topline™ - Scientists keep underestimating the coronavirus. Delta, more than any other variant, has reset scientists' understanding of how quickly a virus can evolve into devastating new forms. Thanks to Delta's infectiousness, and the huge number of people whose refusal or inability to get vaccinated leaves them primed to become living Covid-19 mutation labs, the conditions are ripe to produce yet more, potentially more dangerous, variants in the coming months. Delta is already one of the most transmissible viruses ever encountered, falling short only of the measles. There's anecdotal evidence that more young people are getting severely ill with Delta than has been the case with previous variants. The 1918 flu pandemic preferentially killed younger adults. It's not yet clear whether Delta is hitting the younger harder. Thus far, the vaccines remain highly effective in preventing Delta from causing severe illness leading to hospitalization or death. Fortunately, the virus will at some point run out of ways to become nastier, thanks to the relatively simple structure of the spike protein, which can only be mutated in a few hundred different ways, most of which won't make the virus more harmful.

TMR's Take - The well-researched and lengthy Newsweek article is both alarming and reassuring. It's worth a read. Currently, 1,600 children are hospitalized with Covid-19, Florida Gov. Ron DeSantis has made it illegal for school boards to mandate mask requirements in schools, and the state has the 3rd highest per capita rate of Covid-19 infections in the world behind Louisiana and Botswana. Gov. Greg Abbott's Texas is not far behind, also banning mask mandates. Last century, the comedy duo of Abbott & Costello was frightfully funny; today, the gubernatorial duo of Abbott & DeSantis is just frightening.

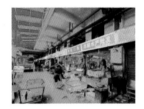

Delayed Wuhan Report Adds Crucial Detail to Covid Origin Puzzle, by Jason Gale, Bloomberg Business Week, 8/23/21

TMR Topline™ - A research study conducted from May 2017 to November 2019 surveying 17 shops at four Wuhan markets selling wild animals remained unpublished until this past June. Conducted by virologist Xiao Xiao, nearly 1/3 of the animals he examined bore trapping and shooting wounds consistent with being caught in the wild, and included masked palm civets, raccoon dogs, bamboo rats, minks and hog badgers. The Huanan market was shuttered 1/1/20, and China's CDC collected specimens that were positive for SARS-CoV-2. A spillover from a wet market in Guangdong caused the 2003 SARS outbreak. In April 2020 a spokesman for China's Foreign Ministry denied that *"wildlife wet markets"* existed in China. Such animals are a well-known path for zoonotic disease transmission.

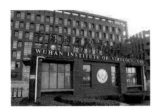

U.S. intelligence agencies delivered a report to Biden on the virus's origins, by Julian E. Barnes, New York Times, 8/25/21

TMR Topline™ - DNI Avril Haines delivered a report to President Biden on the origins of the coronavirus epidemic, but the U.S. spy agencies have not yet concluded whether the disease was the result of an accidental leak from a lab or if it emerged naturally in a spillover from animals to humans. Current and former officials have repeatedly warned that finding the precise origins of the pandemic may be more of a job for scientists than spies. The report remains classified for now. White House Press Secretary Jen Psaki stated *"I can assure you the president wants to get to the bottom of the root causes of Covid-19."*

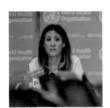

The WHO is looking for experts to help investigate the origins of pathogens — including the coronavirus, by Andrew Joseph, STAT, 8/25/21

TMR Topline™ - The Covid-19 pandemic has elevated scrutiny over how pathogens leap into humans like no crisis before it. To better understand how those events happen, the WHO is setting up a Scientific Advisory Group for the Origins of Novel Pathogens, or SAGO. Maria Van Kerkhove, the agency's technical lead on Covid-19, is seeking up to 25 experts from a range of specialties including biosafety and biosecurity to work with the WHO as new threats arise and previous threats rear up again (e.g., coronaviruses, Lassa, Ebola, avian influenza). The group will help establish frameworks for investigating the origins of pathogens early on as cases of disease are reported, as well as determining the origins of SARS-CoV-2.

TMR's Take - Whodunit? We may never know for certain given China's reluctance to cooperate with international efforts to determine the source of the novel coronavirus. Kudos to the WHO for its proactive response as well as its determination to take politics out of the process and remain rooted in science. As former CDC Director Dr. Thomas Frieden said in his 1/2/21 Wall Street Journal article, Which Countries Have Responded Best to Covid-19? *"Bad politics, quite simply, can trump good public health."* **TMR** wholeheartedly agrees.

CHAPTER 2

Which Countries Protected Their Residents Best?

A S THE NOVEL CORONAVIRUS SPREAD RAPIDLY AROUND THE GLOBE, SOME COUNTRIES RESPONDED IMMEDI-ately and effectively while others stumbled. During the 20 months since the WHO was informed of cases of pneumonia of unknown cause in Wuhan, no country's response has been 100 percent correct 100 percent of the time, but some countries did a far better job of protecting their residents than others.

Surprisingly, some of the world's poorest countries handled the pandemic's onset better than some member nations of the Organization for Economic Cooperation and Development (OECD). In general, the Pacific Rim countries that dealt with the 2003 SARS outbreak and the African countries that were faced with the Ebola threat understood the threat of the novel coronavirus and took measures to contain it.

Among the 37 OECD member nations, initial responses varied widely. In Europe, several countries were caught flat-footed as Covid-19 raged in their care homes. In Belgium, infected residents of eldercare facilities were denied admission to hospitals. According to data compiled by Belgian scientists only 14% of gravely ill residents were admitted to hospitals at the outbreak's peak. Neighboring Germany implemented aggressive testing and contact tracing and practiced social distancing. This worked reasonably well – Germany's per capita fatality rates have consistently been lower than those in France, the U.S., and the U.K. (see chart below). On June 30, 2020, the U.S. per capita fatality rate of 38.6/100,000 ranked 31st of 37 compared with Germany (22) at 10.8, France (32) at 44.6, and the U.K. (36) at 66.1. The OECD average was 26.2/100,000.

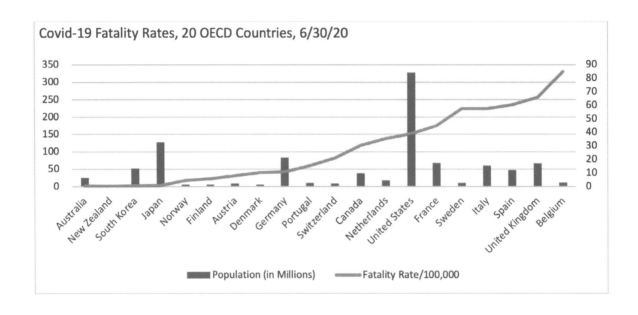

Sweden closed schools for all over-16s and banned gatherings of more than 50, but shops, restaurants and gyms remained open. Although the government now denies it, rumors suggested that the Swedes were attempting to reach "herd immunity," instead attributing Sweden's high fatality rate to deaths that occurred in nursing homes due to shortcomings in eldercare. Meanwhile, its Scandanavian neighbors moved aggressively to combat Covid-19 and have consistently ranked in the first quartile of the OECD.

Covid-19 proved to be a relentless foe.

The eleven weeks from September 20th through November 30th witnessed the rapid rise of Covid-19's second surge, striking ten OECD members in Central Europe with a vengeance (see chart: Fatality Rates, Central Europe, 9/20-11/30/20). Previously, Slovakia had the lowest fatality rate in the Western Hemisphere at 0.72/100,000 thanks to a March 16th national lockdown with universal compliance. Its fatality rate increased twentyfold to 14.67/100,000 by November 30. Likewise, the neighboring Czech Republic experienced a fifteenfold increase from 4.71 to 77.68/100,000. Even Germany, which has maintained the lowest fatality rate among major Western democracies and canceled Oktoberfest, had a 75 percent increase in its fatality rate/100,000 from 11.81 to 19.85.

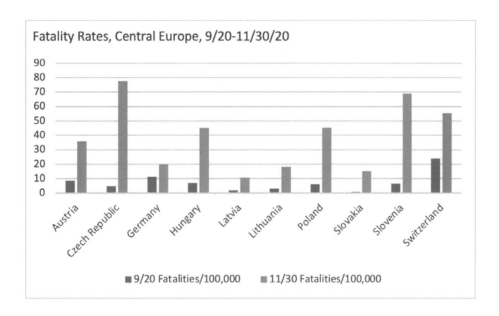

Within the OECD, the Pacific Rim countries, Australia, New Zealand, South Korea and Japan have done an outstanding job of protecting their residents. With fewer ICU beds per capita than hard-hit Italy, New Zealand acted decisively after its first coronavirus case was confirmed on February 28, 2020. On 3/14 Prime Minister Ardern imposed a two-week self-isolation period on anyone entering the country; on 3/19 she banned foreigners from entering the country; and on 3/23 locked down the country of 4.9 million. It worked. By early June, New Zealand had eliminated the novel coronavirus. Fast forward to summer 2021, the highly contagious delta variant invaded the four countries. With low vaccination rates, cases began soaring – even threatening the Tokyo Olympics. Once again, the four countries reacted aggressively and continue to outperform the rest of the OECD (see chart below).

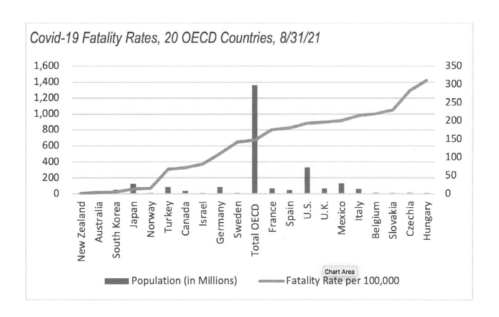

On August 31, 2021, the four major western democracies had moved up significantly in the OECD rankings, with Germany now 15th of 37 with a per capita fatality rate of 110.1/100,000 compared with the OECD average of 147.0/100,000. France was 24th at 175.1, the U.S. 26th at 193.2 and the U.K. 28th at 195.7. Three Central European countries (the Slovak Republic, the Czech Republic and Hungary) had replaced Belgium at the bottom of the barrel.

The 20 article summaries in this chapter provide glimpses at the challenges posed by Covid-19 in 12 countries, some triumphs (e.g., New Zealand, South Korea, Senegal) and some tragedies (e.g., Belgium, India, Hungary), as well as some lessons to be applied in preventing future pandemics.

Pandemic Countries Three Minute Reads

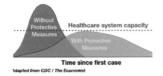

How South Korea Flattened the Curve, by Max Fischer and Choe Sang-Hun, New York Times, 3/24/20

TMR Topline™ - The first Covid-19 cases in America and South Korea were confirmed on January 21. However, South Korea's highest daily new cases occurred on 2/29 (909) and by 3/22 had dropped to 64. How did this country of 50 million succeed in quickly flattening the curve? This article describes the key steps taken to attack the crisis:

1. Intervene fast, before it's a crisis.
2. Test early, often and safely.
3. Implement contact tracing, isolation and surveillance.
4. Enlist the public's help.

TMR's Take - Can their success be replicated in the U.S.? Not exactly. Our diverse population, privacy rules and lack of universal healthcare are barriers. South Korea's single payer system covers at most about 60% of medical bills so nearly 80% of the population also have private insurance. .

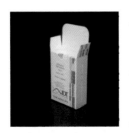

A German Exception? Why the Country's Coronavirus Death Rate Is Low by Katrin Bennhold, New York Times, 4/4/20

TMR Topline™- With a much lower Covid-19 mortality rate (1.8%) than France (9.4%), Spain (9.9%) or Italy (12.6%), this article probes the reasons for Germany's success. The average age of those contracting the disease has been lower (49) than those in France (62.5) and Italy (62), but a key reason for the low fatality rate is that Germany has been testing far more people, catching many with few or no symptoms. Charité Hospital in Berlin developed a test mid-January, posted the formula online and laboratories throughout the country built up a stock of test kits.

Now testing an average of 350,000 patients a week, Germany also has aggressively tracked contacts and practiced social distancing, copying South Korea's strategy. Germany's robust public health system had 28,000 intensive care beds equipped with ventilators (34 per 100,000 people) compared with 12 per 100,000 in Italy and has added capacity since the outbreak.

To many, the "secret sauce" in Germany's low mortality rate has been the leadership of Chancellor Angela Merkel, a scientist by training, who has communicated clearly, calmly and regularly throughout the crisis. Prof. Hans-Georg Kräusslich, head of virology at University Hospital in Heidelberg, summed it up: "Maybe our biggest strength in Germany is the rational decision-making at the highest level of government combined with the trust the government enjoys in the population."

TMR's Take - Germany has had universal healthcare since 1883 and achieved full interoperability in 2008. Medical insurance is mandatory, and Germans can choose from more than 100 not-for profit insurance plans. There is a government buy-in for low income and unemployed. The Eichhorn-Hutchinson Allcare plan has much in common with Germany's time-tested approach to healthcare for all.

Lessons Learned from Lombardy Associated Press, 4/26/20

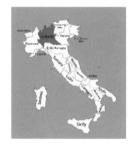

TMR Topline™ - The article provides insights into the perfect storm that slammed the hardest-hit region in Europe's hardest-hit country. With 1/6th of Italy's 60 million people, Lombardy is the most densely populated region, home to the business capital in Milan and Italy's industrial heartland, accounting for 21% of GDP. With the country's highest percentage over 65, Lombardy also has 20% of Italy's nursing homes.

When Italy became the first European country to halt air travel from China on 1/31, it was already too late. Doctors treating patients for pneumonia didn't know it was Covid-19 and were unprepared for many patients rapid decline in the ability to breathe. After years of budget cuts, Italy has only 8.6 ICU beds per 100,000 people, well below the OECD average of 15.9, so many PCPs were treating patients at home, some with supplemental oxygen. Testing was limited by inadequate lab capacity, so PCPs didn't know whether they or their patients were infected. PPE was in short supply and inadequate. A blistering April 7 letter from the doctors' association to regional authorities listed seven errors in their handling of the crisis.

The region's industrial lobbying group resisted shutting down production until 3/26, long after Rome's 3/7 order to shut down Lombardy. Lombardy's nursing homes house more than 24,000 elderly; of 3,045 deaths from 2/1-4/15, 1,625 were either positive for the virus or showed symptoms. A 3/30 regional decree directed nursing homes to not hospitalize sick residents over 75 if they had other health problems. Some nursing homes refused to let staff wear masks to avoid frightening patients. Some local authorities threatened loss of accreditation if the nursing home refused to allow visitors.

TMR's Take - It's little wonder that Lombardy's 73,000 confirmed cases account for 70% of Italy's total.

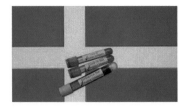

We should have done more, admits architect of Sweden's Covid-19 strategy , by Jon Henley, The Guardian, 6/3/20

TMR Topline™ - With a fatality rate much higher than its Scandinavian neighbors, Anders Tegnell, Sweden's chief epidemiologist, admitted in a radio interview that there was *"quite obviously a potential for improvement in what we have done"* in Sweden. Tegnell had previously been critical of other countries' strict lockdowns as unsustainable in the long run. Sweden closed schools for all over-16s and banned gatherings of more than 50, but shops, restaurants and gyms remained open. Prime Minister Stefan Lovfen defended Sweden's approach as just about right but noted that it had failed to protect care homes where half of all Sweden's Covid-19 deaths have occurred. Its fatality rate of 449 deaths per million was higher than Denmark's (99), Norway's (44) and Finland's (58), but on a par with France and lower than Italy (555), Spain (581) and the U.K. (593).

TMR's Take - It's refreshing to see Sweden's public admission that its pandemic response should have been better. While the U.S. fatality rate was 328 at 5/31, the hard-hit states in the Northeast were much higher: Rhode Island -700; Connecticut – 800; Massachusetts – 1,038; New Jersey – 1,337 and New York – 1,543.

New Zealand has eliminated Coronavirus, Associated Press, 6/8/20

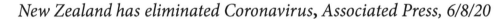

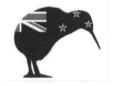

TMR Topline™ - New Zealand health officials announced Monday that the last known infected person had recovered from the coronavirus. With no new cases reported in 17 days, it appears to have completely eradicated the coronavirus -- for now. Prime Minister Jacinda Ardern announced that the Cabinet had agreed to remove almost all remaining virus restrictions except for border restrictions. Over 1,500 people contracted the virus and 22 died, one of the lowest global fatality rates.

TMR's Take - Kudos to the Kiwis! With fewer ICU beds per capita than hard-hit Italy, New Zealand had to act decisively after its first coronavirus case was confirmed 2/28. On 3/14 Prime Minister Ardern imposed a two-week self-isolation period on anyone entering the country; on 3/19 she banned foreigners from entering the country; and on 3/23 locked down the country of 4.9 million.

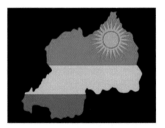

A COVID-19 Success Story in Rwanda: Free Testing, Robot Caregivers, by Jason Beaubien, NPR, 7/15/2020

TMR Topline™ - Mainland Africa's most densely populated country, with per capita income of roughly $2,000 per year, has taken a unique approach to containing Covid-19. Health officials in personal protective equipment administer tests randomly at no cost to the individual. Sample collection and completion of contact information paperwork takes about five minutes. Anyone who tests positive is immediately quarantined at a dedicated Covid-19 clinic. Contact tracing is done and any who are deemed at high risk are quarantined until they can be tested.

Rwanda uses "pool testing" to maximize its testing capacity. If a positive result is obtained, each of the 20-25 nasal swabs are tested individually to identify the infected person(s). Community healthcare workers and police and college students were mobilized to work as contact tracers. Human-size robots are used in the Covid-19 clinics to take patients' temperatures and deliver supplies.

Residents have been following the government's orders regarding masks, washing hands and staying home. The result: the country of 12 million has recorded just over 1,200 cases since its first case in mid-March. With a population of 11.7 million (and four times the area), Ohio has recently been reporting roughly 1,200 cases **a day**.

TMR's Take - A former Belgian colony, Rwanda was the site of a heinous genocide in 1994. What a difference 25 years makes. It's embarrassing to see that a third-world country with limited resources has managed to minimize Covid-19's impact far better than its former parent and the U.S. So much for American exceptionalism.

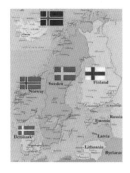

Nordic Study Suggests Open Schools Don't Spread Virus Much, by Kati Pohjanpalo & Hanna Hoikkala, Bloomberg, 7/19/2020

TMR Topline™ - The June 11 issue of **TMR** covered Sweden's failed attempt at reaching "herd immunity." Proof that every cloud may have a silver lining, a Nordic study found that keeping primary schools open during the coronavirus pandemic may not have had much bearing on contagion rates. They found no measurable difference in the number of coronavirus cases among children in Sweden, where schools were left open, compared with neighboring Finland, where schools were shut.

Conducted by the Public Health Agency of Sweden and the Finnish Institute for Health and Welfare, the data showed no difference in the overall incidence of Covid-19 cases in children aged 1-19. Finland's contact tracing found hardly any evidence of children infecting others. A French study recently found that school children don't appear to transmit Covid-19 to peers or teachers, show fewer symptoms than adults, and are less contagious.

Israel's experience was different – the spread of Covid-19 among middle and high school students accelerated after schools reopened. However, Israel has larger class sizes in smaller classrooms. Study co-author Hanna Nohynek, chief physician at the infectious diseases unit of Finland's health authority, said that *"children get sick with Covid-19 much more rarely and less severely."* She cautioned that more data is needed.

TMR's Take - News of the Scandinavian study coincides with Florida's teachers union filing suit to keep the state from reopening its schools for *"at least five days a week for all students,"* while the coronavirus is surging. **TMR** agrees with Dr. Fauci who said the *"default position is that you should try, to the best of your ability, with all considerations to the safety and welfare of the children and the teachers, we should try to get the children back to school as best as we possibly can."*

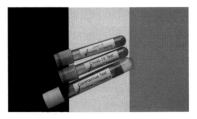

When COVID-19 Hit, Many Elderly Were Left to Die, by Matina Stevis-Gridneff, Matt Apuzzo and Monika Pronczuk, New York Times, 8/9/20

TMR Topline™ - Rapidly spreading infections, lack of PPE and governmental inattention to eldercare facilities have become all too familiar during the global pandemic. However, Belgium's response had an added twist: although hospital ICU beds were available throughout the peak period, hospitals and paramedics sometimes denied care to elderly people. When the pandemic hit northern Italy in February, Maggie De Block, Belgium's federal health minister, played down the risk: *"It isn't a very aggressive virus. You would have to sneeze in someone's face to pass it on,"* adding *"If the temperature rises, it will probably disappear."*

Although government reports had recommended infectious-disease training for nursing home doctors, public help in stockpiling PPE and including nursing homes in the national pandemic plan, the proposals went nowhere. Belgian bureaucracy exacerbated the response: it has nine health ministers who answer to six parliaments. The nursing home situation was so dire that Médecins Sans Frontières dispatched teams of experts in late March. Testing capacity was limited with hospitals taking priority. When nursing home testing finally began April 8 (after more than 2,000 residents already had died), 20% tested positive. At the outbreak's peak only 14% of gravely ill residents were admitted to hospitals according to data compiled by Belgian scientists. The rest were left to receive palliative care. According to University of Antwerp professor Niel Hens, 1,100 of the nation's 2,400 intensive care beds were free at the peak of the pandemic. Ms. De Block has defended the government response stating *"Careful counting, not mismanagement, explains the country's death toll,"* noting with pride that Belgium never ran out of hospital beds.

TMR's Take - Belgium has the highest fatality rate among OECD member nations (85.8/100,000). Its failure to protect its nursing home residents is tragic, accounting for roughly 58% of the country's fatalities, a much higher percentage than in other developed countries.

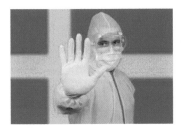

The Swedish COVID-19 Response Is a Disaster. It Shouldn't Be a Model for the Rest of the World, by Kelly Bjorklund and Andrew Ewing, TIME, 10/14/20

TMR Topline™ - Referring to a study published in the Journal of the American Medical Association, the authors argue that Sweden and the U.S. are unique in their failure to reduce coronavirus mortality rates as the pandemic progressed. The table shows fatality rates/100,000 for 7 of 19 high income countries (population > 5,000,000; per capita GDP > $25,000) through 10/13, and from 6/7-10/13. While many countries were hit hard early, Sweden and the U.S. continued to have high fatality rates after 6/7. Sweden's leaders claim success in their efforts to combat the pandemic and deny that their strategy was to build *"herd immunity."* Prime Minister Stefan Löfven and the Public Health Agency attribute Sweden's high Covid-19 death rate to deaths that occurred in nursing homes due to shortcomings in eldercare.

Fatality Rate/100,000 thru 10/13/2020

Country	Start-10/13	6/7-10/13
U.S.	60.3	27.2
Sweden	57.4	10.3
U.K.	62.6	5.0
Spain	65.0	4.6
Belgium	86.8	4.2
France	46.6	3.2
Italy	59.1	3.1

TMR's Take - This thoroughly researched article documents Sweden's failed approach, including not mandating masks or implementing quarantine, even for those returning from travel abroad or family members of those who test positive for Covid-19.

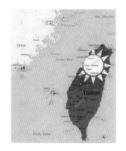

No lockdowns, no downturn: Taiwan attracts skilled expats with (mostly) COVID-free life, by Ralph Jennings and Kim Hjelmgaard, USA TODAY, 11/21/20

TMR Topline™ - Taiwan, a bustling technology hub home to about 24 million people off the coast of southeastern China, is attracting a growing community of expatriates due to its success in controlling the coronavirus. There have been no lockdowns or curbs on economic activity, but masks and fever-checks are ubiquitous. With roughly the same population as Florida, Taiwan has had a total of 607 confirmed cases and seven deaths compared with Florida's more than 897,000 cases and 17,600 deaths. More than 820 entrepreneur residency permits have been approved this year, for example, up from 358 in 2019. Settling in Taiwan does have some downsides – it's densely populated and its English fluency lags Hong Kong and Singapore.

I Am Living in a Covid-Free World Just a Few Hundred Miles From Manhattan, by Stephanie Nolen, New York Times, 11/18/20

TMR Topline™ - Freelance journalist Stephanie Nolan works out at the gym, sends her children to school and gathers friends for dinner without restrictions in virus-free Nova Scotia. A March lockdown included closing provincial borders and even hiking trails. It worked, and restrictions gradually were lifted in June. The pandemic has changed the way people live - social distancing and mask wearing in public are universal. Asked the reasons for the province's success in controlling the virus, Public Health Minister Robert Strang attributed it to public health officials, not politicians, setting policy: "*The message has been that we need to do it to keep each other safe… people accept that.*" Heavily dependent on tourism, the economy has recovered only 80% of the jobs lost in April, businesses have closed, and eviction rates are climbing.

TMR's Take - There is a light at the end of the tunnel, but the new normal will be quite different once the U.S. hunkers down through the next three challenging months.

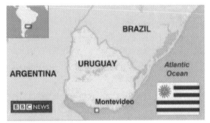

Uruguay to close its borders over holidays due to COVID-19, by Fabian Werner, Hugh Bronstein, Reuters. 12/17/20

TMR Topline™ - Uruguay has closed its borders from Dec. 21 to Jan. 10 except for cargo transportation. Lockdown measures largely held the virus at bay during the first months of the pandemic. "*The second wave to hit the world is our first wave,*" President Luis Lacalle Pou said. Rafael Radi, coordinator of the government's Covid-19 advisory group stated: "*We cannot compromise what has been achieved so far.*"

TMR's Take - Sandwiched between Argentina and Brazil, Uruguay has recorded 174 deaths among its 3.5 million residents for a fatality rate of 5.03/100,000. Elected in March, Lacalle Pou quickly closed borders, instituted widespread testing and contact tracing and appealed for a "*responsible exercise of liberty.*"

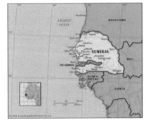

With few resources, Senegal emerges as a leader in the fight against COVID-19, by Fred de Sam Lazaro, NPR, 12/18/20

TMR Topline™ - For much of the pandemic, New Zealand has often been praised for the effectiveness of its response. Despite few resources, the small African nation of Senegal has also become a leader in curbing the Covid-19 pandemic within its borders. This 5-minute video describes how Senegal protected its residents.

TMR's Take –Senegal applied the lessons learned during the Ebola outbreak to protect its 15.9 million residents. At year end its fatality rate was 2.54/100,000. On the African continent, that's behind only Liberia (1.72) and Rwanda (0.68). With a year-end fatality rate of 104.92, COVID-19 has been 50 times deadlier in America than in three of the world's poorest countries.

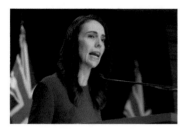

'There's a job to be done': New Zealand's leader explains success against Covid-19, by Associated Press, 12/16/20

TMR Topline™ - New Zealand is the only country to have successfully eliminated the coronavirus. Prime Minister Jacinta Ardern told the AP that the target grew from an early realization the nation's health system simply couldn't cope with a big outbreak. Flattening the curve would not suffice. Border closures and a strict lockdown in March got rid of the disease, and New Zealand went 102 days without any community spread.

An August outbreak in Auckland required a second, more localized lockdown. After winning reelection in an October landslide, Ardern said her job is to build good relationships with every leader and looks forward to working with President-Elect Joe Biden to rebuild New Zealand's relationship with the U.S.

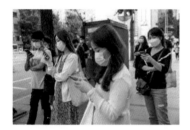

The Country That Learned to Live With Covid-19, Bloomberg, 12/15/20

TMR Topline™ - As nations around the world still struggle to contain Covid-19, South Korea's early, focused, and perhaps controversial approach has kept loss of life and economic damage to a minimum. This 25-minute video provides illuminating insights into the country's success. Its robust contact tracing methods would run afoul of privacy concerns in the U.S. but worked well for South Korea.

TMR's Take - With a population about the same as Italy's and a more densely populated capital city than New York, South Korea confirmed its first Covid-19 case the same day as the U.S. Its test, trace and treat regimen has produced a year-end fatality rate of 1.74/100,000.

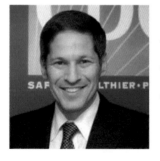

Which Countries Have Responded Best to Covid-19?, by Thomas Frieden MD, Wall Street Journal, 1/2/21

TMR Topline™ - The CDC Director from 2009-17 identifies the countries that, in his opinion, did the best job of responding to the pandemic in 2020:

- Best at early action: Taiwan
- Best at learning from recent epidemics: Liberia (honorable mention - Rwanda and Senegal)
- Best at crushing the curve: New Zealand
- Best at testing: South Korea
- Best at quarantining: Hong Kong
- Best economic protection: Denmark (honorable mention - India, Australia and the EU)
- Best at public communication: Finland (honorable mention - Germany and South Africa)

- Best location in the U.S.: American Samoa (0 deaths from Covid-19, same as 1918-19)

Dr. Frieden noted that many developed countries that did well initially faltered during subsequent surges as their governments and people grew tired of implementing effective strategies. Critical of the U.S. response, he noted that *"Bad politics, quite simply, can trump good public health."*

TMR wholeheartedly agrees.

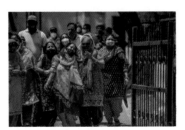

As Covid-19 Devastates India, Deaths Go Undercounted, by Jeffrey Gettleman, Sameer Yasir, Hari Kumar and Suhasini Raj, New York Times, 4/25/21

TMR Topline™ - Months ago, India seemed to have the pandemic under control after a harsh initial lockdown early last year. Now, a second wave is becoming a devastating crisis with more than 300,000 new cases each day and overwhelmed hospitals running out of oxygen.

The sudden surge is casting doubt on India's official Covid-19 death toll of nearly 200,000, with more than 2,000 daily deaths. Bhramar Mukherjee, an epidemiologist at the University of Michigan who has been following India closely said, *"From all the modeling we've done, we believe the true number of deaths is two to five times what is being reported."* Interviews with staff at crematoriums throughout India confirmed that in most cases, they put *"beemari,"* or sickness in Hindi, on all the death certificates, contra to the WHO's rule that the death be recorded as Covid-19-related if the disease is assumed to have caused or contributed to it. Experts say that only about one-fifth of deaths are medically investigated, meaning that the vast number of Indians die without a cause of death being certified. Politics also may play a role. States controlled by Prime Minister Narendra Modi's party may face pressure to underreport, according to some analysts. In 2019, Mr. Modi's government tried to suppress data showing a rise in the unemployment rate.

Equally alarming, India's runaway surge is being driven in part by the emergence of a virus variant known as the *"double mutant,"* B.1.617. One mutation is like the South African variant, the other is like the variant that raged through Southern California, resulting in a variant that is both highly transmissible and more virulent.

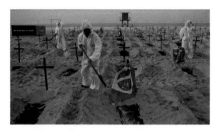

Brazil battles coronavirus with a Chinese vaccine even the Chinese concede could be better, by Heloísa Traiano and Terrence McCoy, The Washington Post, 4/15/21

TMR Topline ™ – Brazil has been using China's CoronaVac vaccine to inoculate its population, only to learn recently that the country was considering changes to its vaccines to *"solve the problem that the efficacy ... is not high."* Brazilian officials have said the vaccine is 78% effective in protecting against moderate and severe covid-19 cases, but 50.4% against all cases. Attempts to control Covid-19 spread have been undone by political divisions, governmental ineptitude, poverty and apathy, and the disease is claiming roughly 3,000 Brazilians a day. Brazilian President Jair Bolsonaro has been skeptical of all vaccines, adding to vaccine hesitancy among the population.

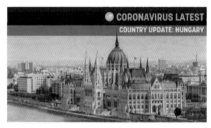

Hungary, despite having one of the world's worst per capita death rates, plans to ease restrictions. by Benjamin Novak, New York Times, 4/1/21

TMR Topline™ - After a month of lockdown measures to combat the virus, Prime Minister Viktor Orban is moving to reopen society. Mass vaccination, he noted, is the only way to bring the suffering to an end, downplaying the death toll and the impact on the nation's struggling hospitals. The independent news media in Hungary is not permitted access to hospitals nor are health care workers allowed to speak with journalists on the record.

TMR's Take - Sadly, the India, Brazil and Hungary articles illustrate again that when politics trump public health, people perish needlessly. At 3/31/21, Hungary's fatality rate of 214.7/100,000 was exceeded only by the Czech Republic among the OECD's 37 members.

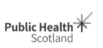

Delta COVID-19 variant doubles risk of hospitalization compared to Alpha strain, Scottish study finds, by Alexandria Hein, Fox News, 6/14/21

TMR Topline™ - The study published 6/14 in The Lancet reported that the Delta variant (B 1.617.2) had become the dominant strain in Scotland and was about twice as likely to result in hospitalization than the Alpha variant (B1.1.7). Conducted from 4/1-6/6/21, the study found that the Delta variant was found mainly in younger, more affluent groups. Fortunately, both the AstraZeneca and Pfizer-BioNTech vaccines cut risk of infection and hospitalization due to the Delta variant, but protection against infection fell as compared with the Alpha variant.

TMR's Take - Heed the doctors lifesaving advice! If you haven't already done so, *get vaccinated!* The life you save may be your own.

CHAPTER 3

With Science Sidelined, U.S. Deaths Surge

THE U.S. RESPONSE TO THE NOVEL CORONAVIRUS WAS SEVERELY HAMPERED BY THEN PRESIDENT TRUMP'S repeated refusal to take responsibility for combating the pandemic. As the first U.S. case was confirmed in Washington state, he consistently played down the threat in public comments and tweets. On January 22nd , he told CNBC *"We have it totally under control. It's one person coming in from China, and we have it under control. It's — going to be just fine,"* subsequently praising China's *"efforts and transparency."*

After the first confirmed U.S. death on February 6th most of the coronavirus messaging from the White House continued to downplay the virus but did set up a task force headed by Vice-President Mike Pence. On February 27th , President Trump predicts: *"It's going to disappear. One day it's like a miracle, it will disappear."* The next day, at a South Carolina rally, he refers to the coronavirus as the Democrats' *"new hoax."* During February, 2.2 million travelers returned from Europe through New York's three airports. Many brought the novel coronavirus with them. As a result, Metro New York joined Milan and Madrid as the global epicenters of the pandemic.

During his March 6th visit to the CDC's Atlanta headquarters, the President stated that *"anybody that wants a test can get a test"* and that he would rather have infected people who were trapped on the Diamond Princess cruise ship stay there to keep the number of confirmed U.S. cases low. Those 13 deaths are listed separately on the Johns Hopkins Coronavirus Resource Center web site and are still excluded from the U.S. total.

On March 11th, the NBA shut down and, in an address from the Oval Office, the President announced a ban on European travel and promised economic relief. By the end of the month, 31 states had implemented various stay-at-home orders. During March, he continually compared the coronavirus to the common flu, a claim debunked by scientific experts. He also claimed incorrectly that the Food and Drug Administration (FDA) approved the antimalarial drug hydroxychloroquine for treating Covid-19.

Congress passed the $2.2 trillion CARES Act March 25, that included direct cash payments for Americans, added funding for hospitals and $500 billion in loans for companies. On March 29th , President Trump extended the CDC's social distancing guidance through April 30, noting *"If we have between 100,000 and 200,000, we've all together done a very good job."* Two days later, he stopped comparing Covid-19 to the seasonal flu, noting that it's *"vicious."*

On April 2nd, President Trump invoked the Defense Production Act to require 3M, Ford, and others to manufacture masks and ventilators. On April 14th, he announces plans to halt funding the WHO, accusing it of *"severely mismanaging and covering up the spread of the coronavirus."* On April 23rd, during a news conference, he suggested injecting bleach as a potential coronavirus treatment.

May 15th saw the announcement of Operation Warp Speed, a public-private partnership to facilitate and accelerate the development and distribution of Covid-19 vaccines, therapeutics and diagnostics. Initially funded with $10 billion from the CARES Act, it is arguably the most effective response to the coronavirus undertaken by the Trump administration. Funding was increased to about $18 billion by October 2020. Companies receiving funding for vaccine development included Johnson & Johnson (Janssen Pharmaceutical), Moderna, Novovax, Astra Zeneca and the University of Oxford, Merck and IAVI, and Sanofi and Glaxo Smith Kline. Pfizer/BioNTech participated in Operation Warp Speed but did not accept any governmental funding.

By May month-end the U.S. death toll had exceeded 100,000.

At June month-end, Covid-19's major impact had been in the Northeast (see chart below).

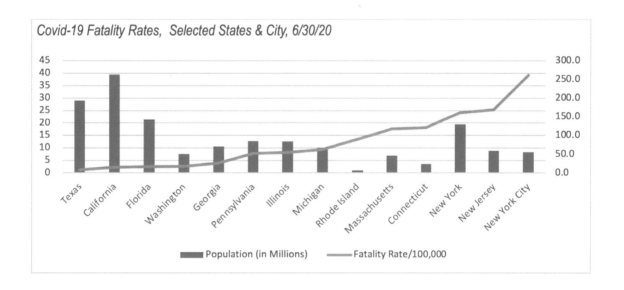

Throughout the year, scientists worldwide were diligently studying Covid-19 to learn how best to prevent, diagnose and treat it. By early Fall, some of their key findings included:

- Airborne transmission is the most dominant route for the spread of Covid-19.
- Loss of the sense of smell (anosmia) is a key indicator of infection.
- Covid-19 hits men harder than women.
- Communities of color are more likely to be vulnerable to infection.
- Obese individuals who contract Covid-19 are more likely to be hospitalized.

- For severe cases where hospitalization is required, where one is treated matters.

- Even in less severe cases, Covid-19's lingering effects are of concern; and

- A supercomputer analysis of more than 2.5 billion genetic combinations has provided a model - the bradykinin hypothesis - that explains many of Covid-19's bizarre symptoms.

Eight months after the first reported case, the U.S. death toll surpassed 200,000 on September 21, roughly equivalent to the population of Salt Lake City or Grand Rapids.

In October, CNBC reported that Health and Human Services Secretary Alex Azar was the keynote speaker at the Goldman Sachs Healthcare virtual event on the coronavirus. He provided an update on the status of vaccine development and manufacturing, noting that Operation Warp Speed expects to have up to 100 million doses by the end of the year, and *We project having enough for every American who wants a vaccine by March to April 2021."* In addition to manufacturing doses for all six potential vaccines backed by the U.S. government across more than 23 manufacturing facilities, the U.S. is also obtaining the needles, syringes, bottles and other supplies needed for immunizations, he said.

On November 9th, Pfizer and its partner, German drug maker BioNTechSE, announced that its Covid-19 vaccine may be 90% effective based on data from its phase 3 clinical trials. One week later, Moderna announced that its experimental vaccine was 94.5% effective in preventing disease, according to an analysis of its clinical trial. Both vaccines consist of genetic material, messenger RNA, encased in tiny particles that shuttle it into cells, then train the immune system to recognize the spiked protein on the surface of the virus. Since it's not made with the coronavirus itself, there's no chance anyone could catch it from the shots.

Both vaccines require two doses for full effectiveness. Pfizer's vaccine requires deep freeze storage but can be kept at refrigerator temperatures for up to five days. The Moderna vaccine can be stored in a freezer and is stable at refrigerator temperatures for up to 30 days.

Both vaccines received emergency use authorization (EUA) from the FDA in early December, and on December 14th , the first doses of the Pfizer/BioNTech were administered. That same day, the U.S. death toll surpassed 300,000, roughly equivalent to the population of St. Louis or Pittsburgh.

The Pfizer/BioNTech rollout encountered some speed bumps and Pfizer CEO Albert Bourla asked the U.S. government to use the Defense Production Act to relieve some *"critical supply limitations."* By January, an average of 3,000 Americans a day were perishing from Covid-19.

On January 19th , the U.S. death toll surpassed 400,000, roughly equivalent to the population of Tampa or Tulsa.

The 26 article summaries in this chapter highlight both the difficult struggles and the hard-won successes in the U.S. efforts to protect its residents from the deadly coronavirus.

Pandemic U. S. 2020 Three Minute Reads

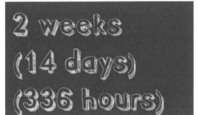

Fourteen Days. That's the Most Time We Have to Defeat Coronavirus, by Ezekiel J. Emanuel, MD, vice provost of global initiatives at the University of Pennsylvania. The New York Times Opinions March 24, 2020

TMR Topline™ - The U.S. must act within the next two weeks to flatten the curve of the Covid-19 pandemic to avoid the dire projections of the Imperial College London model – that up to 2.2 million Americans could die within the next year. While concerned about the economic impact, Dr. Emanuel believes the U.S. economy cannot be restarted without first getting the pandemic under control. To do so, he prescribes five priorities for immediate action.

1. Order all schools and non-essential businesses closed along with a shelter-in-place policy.

2. Accelerate production of test kits and related supplies and remove Covid-19 testing from hospitals and clinics to let them focus on treatment.

3. Appoint a national manufacturing director for the pandemic to assess, allocate and to ramp up production of equipment and disposable supplies.

4. Order hospitals to ban visitors and suspend elective surgeries. Encourage physicians, nurses and other clinicians who are seeing fewer patients because of practice restrictions to work in hospitals. Also, recruit retired and non-practicing physicians, nurses and respiratory therapists to help manage the demand for inpatient coverage.

5. Support small businesses with grants for up to a year to help retain workers and resume operations when the virus is under control.

TMR's Take - To win this war, the U.S. needs to mobilize faster than ever before. Otherwise, Dr. Emanuel warns that it will follow Italy's course and recovery may take a decade or more.

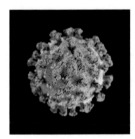

Coronavirus: Things the US has got wrong - and got right BBC News, Anthony Zurcher, North America reporter, 4/1/20

TMR Topline™ - The BBC's North American reporter interviewed numerous experts to paint a clear picture of the shortcomings of the U.S. response as well as some strengths. Zurcher cited the following mistakes:

- Testing delays due to the administration's disregard of pandemic response plans and failure to staff its public health bureaucracy;

- Medical supply shortages (masks, gloves, gowns and ventilators) due both to the government's failure to maintain the stockpile and failure to move quickly when the crisis became apparent;

- Messaging "whiplash" and political squabbles, downplaying the threat during January and February; and
- Social distancing failures like the packed Florida beaches during spring break.

The pandemic has exposed flaws in the U.S. healthcare system including high costs, a lack of universal coverage and supply chains unable to withstand a shock. On a more positive note, Zurcher noted the following successes that will help America to recover:

- Research firepower, with medical researchers and drug companies rushing to learn more about the virus and devise new strategies to defeat the pandemic including rapid-response tests, vaccine development and treatment options;
- State leadership, with governors like Jay Inslee of Washington, Gavin Newsome of California and Mike DeWine of Ohio taking decisive early steps to close schools and issue shelter in place orders; and
- Rapid passage of a massive $2 trillion coronavirus relief bill including direct payments to many Americans, aid to states and healthcare facilities, support for hard-hit industries and loans to small businesses that can be forgiven if they avoid layoffs.

TMR's Take - America's system of government, with broad powers delegated to individual states, has led to a patchwork response that is resulting in avoidable deaths and economic disruption.

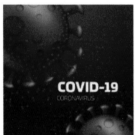

Our Pandemic Summer by Ed Yong, The Atlantic. 4/15/20

TMR Topline™ - Yong lays out the limited options available to the U.S. due to its early inaction. Unlike a hurricane or wildfire, the SARS-CoV-2 virus will linger through the year and across the world. Many ask, "When will it end?" Yong contends that the correct question is "How will we continue?" and suggests four steps:

Reopening. The lockdown has bought the U.S. some time to address its lack of tests and PPE and find less economically devastating ways of controlling Covid-19.

Former FDA commissioner Scott Gottlieb suggests that states should relax their restrictions only after new case counts have fallen for 14 consecutive days. Demand for tests has exploded, but the chemicals needed to complete testing are becoming scarcer. Drugs in short supply rely on interrupted supply chains from China, India and Italy. Add the relentless pressure on exhausted hospital staff and impatience to reopen the country must be tempered.

Recalibration. Yong makes a case for reopening the U.S. slowly and methodically. It is crucial to know what percentage of the population has been infected, to determine which of the social-distancing measures have been most effective, and to do aggressive contact tracing. Then, stay-at-home orders might be the first to be relaxed, but large gatherings are not likely to be allowed until there is an effective vaccine.

Reinforcements. While waiting for a vaccine, medical masks and other PPE must be reserved for those on the frontlines. Effective treatments identified should be used to give critically ill patients a better chance of survival or prevent some people with early symptoms from ever needing critical care at all. Yong details the shortcomings of serological testing, calling instead for *"a modern-day Apollo program."*

Resilience. In his 2018 article questioning whether the U.S. was ready for the next pandemic, Yong noted that we were trapped in a cycle of panic and neglect. He fears that if the current shutdown succeeds in flattening the curve, *"the U.S. might enter the neglect phase before the panic part is even finished."* The success of the mitigation measures in reducing the body count might be used to argue that we overreacted.

TMR's Take - The Covid-19 pandemic is neither a sprint nor a marathon, but an ultra-marathon. The summer ahead will be unusual and the year beyond unsettled.

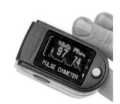

How We Can Get Ahead of COVID-19 Richard Levitan, MD, NY Times, 4/20/20

TMR Topline™ - An emergency medicine physician, Dr. Levitan volunteered to spend 10 days in March at Bellevue Hospital, where he had trained in 1994. Expert in airway management, his "fresh eyes" found Covid pneumonia in patients without respiratory complaints including elderly patients who had passed out for unknown reasons and diabetic patients. X-rays showed moderate to severe pneumonia and low oxygen saturation levels. While most patients had been sick for a week or so with fever, cough, upset stomach and fatigue, they only became short of breath the day they came to the hospital. Their *"silent hypoxia"* resulted in arriving at the hospital in critical condition. Normal oxygen saturation is 94-100%; Covid pneumonia patients had oxygen saturations as low as 50 percent.

TMR's Take - The SARS-CoV-2 virus is insidious and its course devastating. Use of a pulse oximeter in addition to monitoring for fever can detect Covid pneumonia early in the disease's course.

National Action Plan for Expanding and Adapting the Healthcare System for the Duration of the COVID Pandemic Johns Hopkins Bloomberg School of Public Health, Center for Health Security, 5/5/20

TMR Topline™ - This report from the experts at Johns Hopkins is a thoughtful examination of key shortcomings that the pandemic has brought to light, along with 47 recommendations for addressing them while U.S. healthcare continues the battle. Summarized below are the ten problems addressed in the report along with some of the recommendations.

How can we improve infection prevention in hospitals and maintain a robust supply chain for personal protective equipment (PPE)? Healthcare facilities should develop crisis standard of care plans for PPE and the federal government should create a centralized information-sharing system so that, in a declared emergency, states and healthcare facilities work collaboratively in sourcing PPE and other scarce medical supplies.

What approach should we take to restarting deferred healthcare services? Resumption of deferred inpatient and outpatient services should be prioritized (triaged) based on an assessment of objective patient health needs and availability of needed hospital space, equipment, supplies, and staff.

What financial support is needed for hospitals and healthcare providers? HHS should determine how much additional funding may be needed to cover health-sector losses due to the pandemic and consider establishing a crisis fund to provide short-term bridge funding for hospitals on the verge of financial collapse.

How should the healthcare workforce be sustained and augmented? Regulatory constraints addressing licensure, certification, and scope of practice of healthcare workers need to be relaxed to augment the existing healthcare workforce, and existing regulatory barriers to telephone- or video-based clinical encounters should be removed.

How can we provide mental health support for healthcare workers in this crisis? Hospitals and other providers should make counseling available to staff and implement mental health and well-being support programs. Local and state governments should consider jurisdiction-wide mental health support programs for healthcare workers.

How can we provide medical care and sick leave for all people in the United States? Given the high and growing number of uninsured people in the country due to this crisis, Congress should develop a plan to ensure access to affordable healthcare coverage for all Americans.

How can we make telemedicine a new normal? Payers should reimburse telemedicine visits on par with in-person visits.

How can we reduce the number of undiagnosed infectious diseases in our hospitals? CMS and other payers should separate diagnostic testing from bundled payments.

How can we better protect emergency medical services (EMS) personnel from infectious diseases? Federal, state, and local governments should prioritize and fund EMS systems and providers to receive PPE, particularly N95 respirators, on par with hospitals. Longer term, CMS should reconsider the reimbursement process for EMS, and state and local governments should reassess the baseline funding needs of EMS.

How can we better coordinate the healthcare response to Covid and the next pandemic? Electronic medical records must be made interoperable, more accessible, and searchable by public health personnel to aid in state and federal situational awareness and emergency management.

TMR's Take - The 24-page report should be required reading for anyone interested in preparing the healthcare system to deal more effectively with the next pandemic. Healthcare already was the #1 issue on voters' minds before the Covid-19 pandemic arrived. Will Congress have the political will to place public health above politics and invest hundreds of billions to avoid a multi-trillion hit to the economy? Stay tuned.

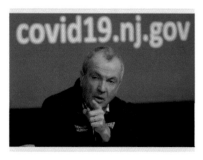

N.J. governor unveils proposal on improving nursing home outbreak response Modern Healthcare, 6/4/20

TMR Topline™ - New Jersey's long-term care facilities experienced disproportionately high Covid-19 fatality rates. In responding to the outbreak, the state commissioned a review by Manatt Health's experts to look at what added protocols, resources and equipment should be put in place to best protect the residents. The report was released 6/3. Key recommendations include:

- Strengthen Emergency Response Capacity by strengthening the ability to plan, coordinate, and execute effective responses to the emergency protentional surges.

- Stabilize Facilities and Bolster Workforce by increasing the responsibilities of and support for New Jersey's nursing homes and their workers in the short and long-term.

- Increase Transparency and Accountability by implementing stronger mechanisms to ensure a greater degree of accountability and increase transparency through data and reporting.

- Build a More Resilient and Higher Quality System by establishing structures for stronger collaboration and advance payment and delivery reforms and increased reliance on home and community-based services.

The report did not address why New Jersey's case volume and fatality rates were so much higher than other states.

TMR's Take - Long-term care facilities are sitting ducks when a highly contagious and potentially lethal virus is unleashed. Kudos to New Jersey for its proactive response to identify corrective measures that may serve as a template for others. The Legislature will be investigating the high case volumes and fatality rates.

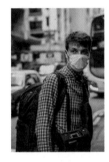

Community Use Of Face Masks And COVID-19, by Wei Lyu and George L. Wehby, Health Affairs, 6/16/20

TMR Topline™ - While the WHO recommends that symptomatic individuals wear face masks in public, there has been an ongoing debate as to whether asymptomatic individuals also should do so. On April 3, the CDC issued new guidance advising all individuals to wear cloth facial covers in public areas where close contact with others is unavoidable, citing new evidence on virus transmission from asymptomatic individuals.

This study provides direct evidence on the effects of state government mandates in the U.S. for face mask use in public issued by 15 states plus DC between April 8th and May 15th. It estimates that as many as 230,000–450,000 Covid-19 cases may have been averted based on when states passed these mandates. The authors conclude: "*As countries worldwide and states begin to relax social distancing restrictions and considering the high likelihood of a second Covid-19 wave in the fall/winter, requiring use of face masks in public might help in reducing Covid-19 spread.*"

TMR's Take - This study confirms the effectiveness of wearing face masks in public as a mitigation measure. Prudence suggests that the U.S. should join Germany, France, Italy, Spain, China, and South Korea in mandating the wearing of face masks in public.

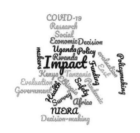

Impact of Coronavirus on Personal Health, Economic and Food Security, and Medicaid, Kaiser Family Foundation, 5/27/20

TMR Topline™ - The KFF's monthly tracking poll had some disturbing results: Nearly half of adults (48%) say they or someone in their household have postponed or skipped medical care due to the coronavirus outbreak. Another 39% say worry or stress related to coronavirus has had a negative impact on their mental health while 31% say they have fallen behind in paying bills or had problems affording household expenses. Most adults (55%) say the Medicaid program is personally important to them and their families.

TMR's Take - The KFF is a trusted source for credible information and the May survey results are disturbing. **TMR** will continue to monitor.

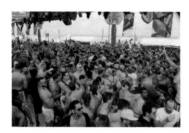

Parties — Not Protests — Are Causing Spikes in Coronavirus, by Christiana Silva, NPR, 6/24/20

TMR Topline™ - NPR's report from Washington state found that despite drawing massive crowds, protests against police violence and racial injustice in Washington state weren't among the clusters where multiple people contracted Covid-19 at the same event or location. Using contact tracing, local officials found that 14 cases (and a subsequent 15 more) were associated with a party of 100 to 150 people in early June. When asked about protests in Bellingham, the County Health Department Director Erika Lautenbach told NPR's *All Things Considered*: "*Almost everyone at the rally was wearing a mask, and it's really a testament to how effective masks are in preventing the spread of this disease.*"

TMR's Take - Two articles summarized in the prior issue spoke to the effectiveness of wearing face masks in public as a mitigation measure. Whatcom County's contact tracing provides independent validation. The National Bureau of Economic Research recently released "Black Lives Matter Protests, Social Distancing, and COVID-19," which examined protests in 315 of the largest U.S. cities and found "*no evidence that urban protests reignited Covid-19 case growth during the more than three weeks following protest onset.*"

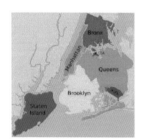

Why Surviving Covid Might Come Down to Which NYC Hospital Admits You, by Brian M. Rosenthal, Joseph Goldstein, Sharon Otterman and Sheri Fink, The New York Times, 7/1/20

TMR Topline™ - This investigative article found significant disparities in care between hospitals in Manhattan compared with those in the outer boroughs. Manhattan is home to many world-renowned medical centers serving insured patients while the outer boroughs are served by a patchwork of satellite campuses, city-run public hospitals and independent facilities with higher volumes of Medicare, Medicaid and uninsured patients. At the 11 public safety net hospitals only 10% of patients have private insurance.

Manhattan has 5.0 beds per 1,000 residents compared with 1.8 in Queens, 2.2 in Brooklyn and 2.4 in the Bronx. Interviews with clinicians on the front lines during the crisis detail the lack of adequate staff and equipment to deal with the tsunami of Covid-19 patients. At Mount Sinai's flagship hospital, 17% of such patients died, compared with 33% at its Queens campuses and 34% its Brooklyn campuses. Hospital executives objected to the use of raw mortality data, contending that it was meaningless unless adjusted for patients age and underlying conditions.

TMR's Take - Covid-19's disproportionate impact on Black and Latino communities has been widely recognized. However, the Times investigative story raises the issue that the place of treatment also has a major effect on mortality rates.

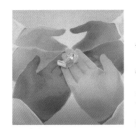

'If I Hadn't Been Transferred, I Would Have Died', By Daniela J. Lamas, New York Times, 8/4/20

TMR Topline™ - A critical care doctor at Boston's Brigham and Women's Hospital, Dr. Lamas uses the story of a patient's successful recovery to illustrate the complexities of critical care medicine in coping with the challenges of Covid-19. After more than three weeks on the ventilator and a stay at the long-term rehab hospital where she rebuilt the strength to walk again, her patient recently had run four miles four months after being diagnosed. The sickest patients who survived required meticulous critical care, combining resources and competency available in only a handful of hospitals.

JAMA Internal Medicine recently published a large study that examined mortality rates for more than 2,200 critically ill coronavirus patients in 65 hospitals throughout the country and found that patients admitted to hospitals with fewer than 50 ICU beds were three times more likely to die. An earlier investigative piece in The Times found that at the peak of the pandemic, patients at some community hospitals were three times more likely to die than patients in medical centers in wealthier areas. During a video visit, Dr. Lamas' patient reminded her that she was initially admitted to a small hospital in western Massachusetts, noting *"If I hadn't been transferred, I would have died."* Dr. Lamas recommends devoting resources to helping hospitals deliver high-quality critical care, perhaps through a more coordinated system of hospital-to-hospital patient transfers within each region to a coronavirus center of excellence.

TMR's Take –Even after a safe, effective vaccine is available, Americans will continue to contract Covid-19 with many becoming seriously ill. With the pandemic now raging in rural America, time is of the essence – among rural hospitals in 20 states, 66% lack ICU beds.

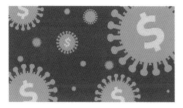

COVID-19 long-term toll signals billions in healthcare costs ahead, by Caroline Humer, Nick Brown; Emilio Parodi and Alistair Smout; Reuters, 8/3/20

TMR Topline™ - There is mounting evidence that some Covid-19 survivors face months and possibly much longer periods of debilitating complications from the virus. These symptoms include breathing difficulties, neurological issues, heart complications, kidney disease and motor skill problems.

Bruce Lee of the City University of New York, Public School of Health estimates that if 20% of the U.S. population contracts this virus, the one-year cost could be $50 billion. Dr. Lee estimates that the annual cost of care for a patient that has been hospitalized with the virus is $4,000 and he also estimates the cost of care for patients who were not hospitalized at $1,000 per year. These costs can vary widely depending on the type of care that the patient may require. For example, Anne McKee a retired psychologist who lives in the southeast, has spent more than $5,000 on doctors' visits and prescriptions over the last five months since she contracted the virus. During this period her insurance company has paid more than $15,000 for her care.

The United Kingdom plans to track the health status of 10,000 patients who have been hospitalized with Covid-19 for as long as 25 years to define the characteristics of the long-term Covid-19 syndrome as they have done with Ebola survivors in Africa.

TMR's Take - Like other viruses, Covid-19's effects will linger long after the initial encounter, even among younger patients with mild symptoms. Dr. Anthony Fauci recently said post-viral Covid-19 syndrome is fast becoming a patient care problem: *"Brain fog, fatigue and difficulty in concentrating, so this is something we really need to seriously look at.*

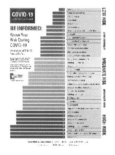

You've Checked Your Temperature. Now, What's Your Risk Tolerance?, by Elizabeth Rosenthal, MD, New York Times, 8/19/20

TMR Topline™ - Tired of hearing people say, *"I'm not going back to life until there's a vaccine,"* Dr. Rosenthal challenges Americans to take stock of their risk tolerance. Noting that outbreaks of polio, mumps, measles and chickenpox were prevalent until vaccines were developed, she provides examples from her experience as a New York City emergency room physician and at a coastal clinic in Kenya. Accepting risk means taking precautions and deciding that you can live with the reduced risk that remains. Dr. Rosenthal urges that masking be mandated and enforced. In addition to wearing a mask and social distancing when not at home, avoid prolonged periods in indoor spaces with crowds or strangers; wash or sanitize hands frequently and avoid "high touch" surfaces.

TMR's Take - The coronavirus is here to stay. Those at high risk for infection need to take precautions, but most Americans will find Dr. Rosenthal's advice reasonable.

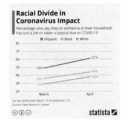

The Coronavirus Race Gap, Explained, by Jeneen Interlandi, New York Times, 10/4/20

TMR Topline™ - Black and Latino Americans are roughly two to three times more likely to contract the coronavirus, four times more likely to be hospitalized and three times as likely to die from it. The CDC found that 80% of the 121 children who died by the end of July were children of color. NPR also analyzed Covid-19 demographic data collected by the Covid Racial Tracker. The review found that in 32 states plus Washington D.C., Black Americans are dying at rates higher than their proportion of the population. In 21 states, it's more than 50% above what would be expected. Likewise, Latinos and Hispanics test positive for the coronavirus at rates twice as high as would be expected for their share of the population in 30 states.

Many low-income workers who are essential to the economy are persons of color who can't work from home. They are the transit, farm and food plant workers, the nursing home aides and cashiers and delivery people that go to work each day. Many have other risk factors such as poor nutrition, inadequate health care, and crowded housing, making them more vulnerable to the virus and its worst effects. Americans of color have faced higher rates of chronic illness and infant mortality for generations. Doctors and public health experts have worked to address these disparities, says Margaret Handley, an epidemiologist at the University of California, San Francisco. They are determined to use the coronavirus crisis to forge meaningful progress against this disparity of access to care for minorities. *"If one good thing comes out of Covid, it may be that we finally build the momentum to do this,"* Dr. Handley said.

Alicia Fernandez, a primary care doctor at Zuckerberg San Francisco General Hospital, suggests that if you want to stop the coronavirus from working its way through factories and farms, these workplaces should be unionized. Dr. Fernandez believes that unions could make a difference, stating *"Data shows that for nursing home workers, being in a union was associated with better protection and less infections."* The United Farm Workers Foundation reports that 99% of all farm workers are not unionized. They are less likely to receive masks and other protective gear from their employers, less likely to be informed about outbreaks where they work and more likely to face retaliation if they voice concerns.

The Congressional Hispanic Caucus recently held a panel discussion on this issue with doctors and other healthcare professionals. The lawmakers wanted to know what was being done to curb the imbalance of Covid infection and care among Latinos and Blacks. When a vaccine becomes available, who would ensure that community health centers serving large numbers of Black and Latino patients would receive an adequate supply, and what could be done to combat vaccine hesitancy? Whether the existing racial health gap expands or contracts, depends in part on the answer to such questions. Said on caucus member, *"We are all facing the same storm, but we are not all in the same boat."*

TMR's Take - Universal access to affordable healthcare for all Americans would reduce inequality in healthcare, addressing the race gap issue that the pandemic has brough to light.

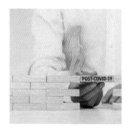

Post-COVID Clinics Get Jump-Start From Patients With Lingering Illness, by Julie Appleby, Kaiser Health News, 9/30/20

TMR Topline™ - More than 7 million Americans have survived Covid-19, but many continue to wrestle with a range of physical or mental effects, including lung damage, heart or neurological concerns, anxiety and depression. Researchers estimate that 10% of recovered patients may have long-lasting symptoms.

Major health systems are starting post-Covid clinics that bring together medical professionals from a range of specialties, including physicians who specialize in lung disorders, heart issues and brain and spinal cord problems. Mental health specialists are also involved, along with social workers and pharmacists. There are about a dozen such clinics nationally, including at Mount Sinai Medical Center in New York City, with more than 400 patients enrolled thus far. By providing more cost-effective, coordinated care that avoids duplicative testing, such multi-specialty post-Covid clinics could help lower health spending and provide a new revenue source for hospitals.

TMR's Take - Post-Covid clinics are not likely to become the next cardiac rehab centers but could add a needed revenue source for major teaching hospitals while benefitting *"long haulers"* whose symptoms linger after recovering from the initial Covid-19 infection.

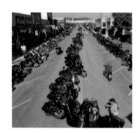

How the Sturgis Motorcycle Rally may have spread coronavirus across the Upper Midwest, by Brittany Shammas and Lena H. Sun, Washington Post, 10/17/20

TMR Topline™ - Despite the concerns expressed by health experts ahead of the event, the annual Sturgis Motorcycle Rally drew nearly 500,000 to the small South Dakota town from August 7-16. Rallygoers filled bars, restaurants, concert venues and tattoo parlors with many going unmasked. By mid-September, more than 330 cases and one death were causally linked to the rally. The Dakotas, along with Wyoming, Minnesota and Montana, were leading the nation in new coronavirus infections per capita. Experts agree that the total number of cases will never be known since contact tracing doesn't always capture the source of the infection and asymptomatic spread goes unnoticed. Kaiser Family Foundation epidemiologist Josh Michaud said: *"Holding a half-million-person rally in the midst of a pandemic is emblematic of a nation as a whole that maybe isn't taking [the novel coronavirus] as seriously as we should."*

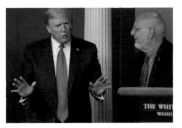

A new study finds poor leadership is the reason for America's unrivaled coronavirus death toll, by Hilary Brueck, Business Insider, 10/21/20

TMR Topline™ - Citing data from the same JAMA study as the Swedes, Brueck makes the case that *"The U.S. did not ever sufficiently put its guard up against this virus at the federal level,"* and it now leads the world in pandemic death rates. Since June, no other large rich country has fared as poorly as the U.S. (see chart, below). Even Belgium, that is highest in the OECD fatality rate resulted from its negligence of its care home population, crushed the curve. The U.S. fatality rate since 6/7 is roughly five times France and four times Spain and Sweden. Only Mexico and Brazil have fatality rates on a par with the U.S. Study co-author Ezekiel Emanuel stated: *"We lacked federal leadership and coordination that we needed."*

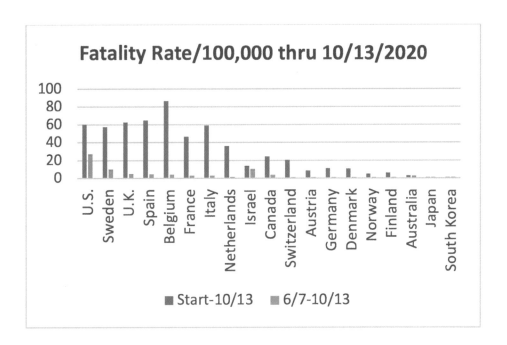

Emanuel and other public health experts agree that until there are treatments and approved vaccines, defeating the pandemic virus requires a better coordinated public health response from state to state, and better nationwide disease surveillance.

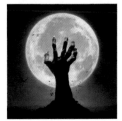

TMR's Take - The song lyrics say it best: *"Blue moon, you saw me standing alone."* Once again, America is the disgrace of the developed world with the highest per capita fatality rate in the OECD. The Editor's 2016 series of articles in Garden State Focus documented American healthcare as the worst value in the developed world. Part 2 of his current series, "The COVID-19 Pandemic – How is the U.S. Doing?" was published earlier this month. Its opening line: *"The short answer – not well."*

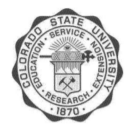

The Best COVID Warning System? Poop and Pooled Spit, Says One Colorado School, by Rae Allen Michell, Kaiser Health News, 11/3/20

TMR Topline™ - With more than 23,000 undergraduates on its Fort Collins campus, Colorado State University has been more successful in combating community spread than the somewhat bigger University of Colorado at Boulder. How? By scanning the contents of undergraduates' feces extracted from 17 manholes connected to dorm buildings early each morning. The sewage review is part of a multipronged attack that includes contact tracing plus a specialized *"paired pooling"* form of testing saliva samples. Emerging research shows that infected people start shedding the coronavirus in their poop days before they begin shedding it from their mouths and noses. Carol Wilusz, a CSU molecular biologist, said *"We can catch them before they're actually spreading the infection."*

CSU also figured out how to screen saliva for less than $20 a person compared with the $93/test using the nose swab method. It involves pooling drool samples in a strategic way reminiscent of the children's game Battleship. They start with an eight-by-eight grid of saliva from 64 people, arrayed almost like a Battleship board. Each person's spit sample gets divided up and analyzed in two pools, one pool for the row it sits in and one for the column it sits in, for a grand total of 16 pools per grid. If the test containing samples in Row A and the test containing samples from Column One appear positive, that would indicate that the person whose spit is in the A-1 slot is a positive case.

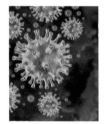

Studies show drop in COVID death rate, by Caitlin Owens, Axios, 10/21/20

TMR Topline™ - Two new peer-reviewed studies have confirmed a sharp drop in mortality rates among hospitalized Covid-19 patients. In one study, researchers looked at more than 5,000 hospitalizations in the NYU Langone health system between March and August. After adjusting for age and underlying conditions, patients in the study had a 25.6% chance of dying at the start of the pandemic; they now have a 7.6% chance. A study of 21,000 hospitalized cases at the Alan Turing Institute in the U.K. also found a similarly sharp drop in the death rate. Both studies attributed the decline to developing more standardized treatments for the virus as well as getting better at identifying when patients are at risk of blood clots or a severe immune system reaction. Wearing masks may be helping as infected individuals receive less of an initial dose of the virus.

A study released by the CDC found that hospitalized patients with Covid-19 in the Veterans Health Administration had a more than five times higher risk for in-hospital death than those suffering from the flu. The study also found that the risks for complications of Covid-19 were higher among non-Hispanic Black or African American and Hispanic patients than among non-Hispanic White patients

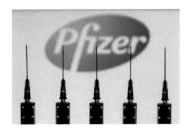

Five Questions to Ask About Pfizer's Covid-19 Vaccine, by Arthur Allen, Kaiser Health News, 11/10/20

TMR Topline™ - Pfizer's mRNA based Covid -19 vaccine developed with BioNTech appears to keep nine of 10 people from getting the disease. If so, it's a breakthrough with a whole new class of vaccines. Five critical questions must be answered to be confident that this vaccine should be broadly distributed and injected:

1. **How long will the vaccine protect patients?** Of nearly 40,000 in the trial, 94 got ill, but Pfizer didn't indicate how long protection will last or how often boosters might be needed.

2. **Will it protect the most vulnerable?** The demographics of the volunteers who received the vaccine was not disclosed.

3. **Can it be rolled out effectively?** It must be kept supercooled at -100F. Pfizer has developed a system to transport the vaccine in specially designed cases to vaccination sites but mishandling the vaccine from manufacture to patient would render it ineffective.

4. **Could a premature announcement hurt future vaccines?** Quick approval by the FDA could make it harder for other manufacturers of vaccines to complete their studies. More trials are important as many vaccines will be needed to meet the global demand.

5. **Could the Pfizer study expedite future vaccines?** Scientists are interested in whether those who received the vaccine but still got sick produced lower levels of antibodies than those who remained well. This would help public health officials to determine if other vaccines under production were effective without having to test them on tens of thousands of people.

Former FDA Deputy Commissioner Dr. Joshua Sharfstein said: *"I hope this makes people realize that…there's hope coming, whether it's this vaccine or another."*

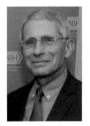

Dr. Fauci says COVID-19 vaccine could be widely available by April, by Brittany Bowker, Boston Globe, 11/10/20

TMR Topline™ - Interviewed by Jake Tapper on CNN, Dr. Anthony Fauci stated that vaccinations must go through a *"tried and true"* process of prioritization and the Pfizer vaccine could be available to everyone by April 2021. He anticipates health providers will be the highest priority for the vaccine, followed by people with *"underlying comorbidities"* that put them at high risk for serious infection, followed by the elderly. In an NBC interview, Dr. Fauci said *"I trust Pfizer and the FDA… if they say this data is solid, then I promise I will take the vaccine and I recommend that my family take the vaccine."*

TMR's Take –Much progress has been made despite the speed bumps encountered in America's scattershot response to the pandemic. Even at lower mortality rates, Covid-19 is five times deadlier than the seasonal flu, so wash your hands, wear a mask and socially distance.

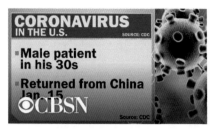

Coronavirus Was In U.S. Weeks Earlier Than Previously Known, Study Says by Jaclyn Diaz, NPR, 12/1/20

TMR Topline™ - The first Covid-19 case in the US was confirmed on Jan.20, a traveler returning from China. However, SARS-CoV-2 infections may have been present in the U.S. in December 2019. The CDC analyzed blood donations collected by the American Red Cross between Dec. 13 and Jan. 17 from residents in nine states. Researchers found coronavirus antibodies in 39 samples from California, Oregon, and Washington as early as Dec. 13 to Dec. 16 as well as in 67 samples from Connecticut, Iowa, Massachusetts, Michigan, Rhode Island, and Wisconsin in early January. The findings were reported in the journal *Clinical Infectious Diseases.* The authors concluded *"These findings also highlight the value of blood donations as a source for conducting SARS-CoV-2 surveillance studies."*

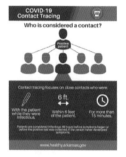

Where COVID Is on the Menu: Failed Contact Tracing Leaves Diners in the Dark, by Anna Almendrala, Kaiser Health Network, 12/1/20

TMR Topline™ - Restaurants appear to be among the most common places to get infected with Covid-19 but contact tracing in most areas has been so lackluster that few health departments have been able to link disease clusters to in-person dining. Covid-19 spreads mainly through respiratory droplets that an infected person can release by sneezing, coughing, or talking. Dining inside a restaurant combines several high-risk activities including removing one's mask to eat and drink, and dining with people from outside one's household. Meals served indoors presents larger risks since the virus has the potential to linger in still air.

A ten state study by the CDC found that those who had tested positive for Covid-19 were more than twice as likely to say they had dined in a restaurant in the two weeks before beginning to feel sick, compared with those who tested negative. Dining out was the only significantly different activity between those who tested positive and those who tested negative. The study found no increased risk of infection linked to shopping, gathering with ten or fewer people or spending time in an office. In Houston, 8.7% of Covid-positive people interviewed for tracing listed a restaurant, cafe or diner as a potential source of exposure since the beginning of June.

Restaurant restrictions have proven to be effective at slowing viral spread in a community. Of the many mitigation measures that states implemented at the beginning of the pandemic, shutting down restaurants had the strongest correlation to reducing the spread of the disease, according to researchers at the University of Vermont. A recent Stanford University-led study that used mobile phone data from different cities to create a simulation of viral spread suggests that restaurants operating at full capacity spread four times as many additional Covid-19 infections as the next-worst location, indoor gyms.

KHN contacted 25 health departments in America's most populous counties. Only nine were collecting and reporting data on potential links between restaurants and Covid-19 cases. Priority often is given to learning the names of individuals over the locations where the coronavirus may be spreading. Many countries have succeeded in following individual trails of virus. In Japan, investigators use contact tracing to identify clusters of disease. Of about 3,000 cases confirmed from January to April, investigators identified 61 clusters, 16% of which were in restaurants or bars.

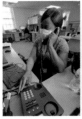
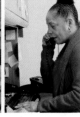

Why shame and fear are hurting N.J.'s battle against COVID-19, by Rebecca Everett, Star-Ledger, 12/7/20

TMR Topline™ - Of the Covid-19 positive people contact tracers are reaching, they're only sharing information about their exposures about half the time. And when it comes to giving out their close contacts' information, only about 30% are cooperating. People are often reluctant to tell contact tracers where they've been because it may involve admitting that they did something they've been told not to, like going to a party or other gathering without masks. Perry Halkitis, dean of The School of Public Health at Rutgers University, suggests that more sophisticated messaging could help.

TMR's Take - Deployed effectively, contact tracing is one of the most powerful weapons in battling a pandemic. However, it requires cooperation from the public and identifying clusters of viral spread. Shame and its cousin guilt can contribute to people's reluctance to cooperate with contact tracers. That's just basic human nature.

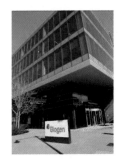

Boston conference in February linked to as many as 300,000 coronavirus cases worldwide, by Morgan Gstalter, The Hill, 12/11/20

TMR Topline™ - The 175 attendees at Biogen's 2/27-28 international business conference in Boston have been linked to as many as 300,000 coronavirus cases worldwide according to a study published in Science. Lead author Jacob Lemieux, an infectious disease specialist at Massachusetts General Hospital, used the virus's unique genetic signature to link it to Covid-19 cases in several countries and 29 states, including about 71,450 cases in Florida.

TMR's Take - And all along we thought it was Spring Break that started the Sunbelt's summer surge.

CHAPTER 4

Biden Takes Office, Declares War on Covid-19 – is the U.S. Winning?

O N THE EVE OF HIS INAUGURATION, PRESIDENT JOE BIDEN PAID TRIBUTE TO THE 400,000 AMERICANS WHO perished from Covid-19. Four-hundred lights around the Lincoln Memorial's reflecting pool were lit and both he and Vice-President Elect Kamala Harris spoke. At his inauguration, Biden asked for a moment of silent prayer stating: *"We're entering what may be the toughest and deadliest period of the virus and must set aside politics and finally face this pandemic as one nation."*

He wasted no time attacking the pandemic. That afternoon, his first three Executive Orders targeted Covid-19: requiring masks on federal property, rejoining the World Health Organization and establishing a White House Covid-19 response team led by Jeff Zients. The series of orders and presidential directives that Biden signed were aimed at jump starting his national Covid-19 strategy to increase vaccinations and testing, lay the groundwork for reopening schools and businesses, and immediately increase the use of masks. Promising stringent adherence to public health guidance, Biden declared: *"To a nation waiting for action, let me be clear on this point: help is on the way."*

More than 97,000 Americans died from Covid-19 during January bringing the cumulative death toll to more than 440,000. The U.S. per capita fatality rate of 134.5/100,000 ranked 32nd out of the 37 OECD member nations, trailed only by Italy, the Czech Republic, the U.K., Slovenia and Belgium. To put the death toll in context, 416,800 Americans died during the 45 months of World War Two.

President Biden's initial goal of administering 100 million vaccine doses in his first 100 days was reached on day 58, and more than 200 million doses were administered by day 100. On February 27, the Food and Drug Administration issued an emergency use authorization (EUA) for Johnson & Johnson's single dose adenovirus vaccine, further expanding the availability of safe effective vaccines for Covid-19. The vaccine was 72% effective in the US, compared to 66% in Latin America and 57% in South Africa. Unlike the Pfizer/BioNTech and

Moderna mRNA-based vaccines, J&J's Janssen vaccine requires only one injection and can be stored for at least three months at 36-46F.

With a moment of silence and a candlelit memorial, President Biden marked the loss of life from Covid-19, as the U.S. death toll surpassed 500,000 on February 22nd , roughly equivalent to the population of Kansas City, Missouri

The $1.9 trillion American Rescue Plan Act (ARPA) was signed into law on March 11th , the one-year anniversary of the WHO's declaration of Covid-19 as a global pandemic. Not a single Republican in either the House or the Senate voted for the bill. It contains the most extensive health insurance improvements for Americans since the Affordable Care Act (ACA) became law 11 years ago.

The ARPA temporarily extends the eligibility criteria for ACA subsidies to include people with incomes above 400% of the federal poverty level so that no one must pay more than 8.5% of their income on insurance premiums. The Congressional Budget Office estimates that the ACA changes will extend coverage to 2.5 million uninsured Americans. The federal government will cover 100% of COBRA premiums for laid-off workers between April 1st and September 30th . The ARPA also offers two years of additional federal funding to encourage Medicaid expansion in the 12 states that have not extended coverage to low-income adults.

The ARPA also contains important provisions to deal with the economic consequences of the pandemic, including $1,400 stimulus checks, expansion of the child tax credit, support for low-income families and childcare facilities, and rent support. Economists estimate that the poorest fifth of Americans will experience a more than 20 percent increase in their incomes. It should reduce poverty by one-third, reducing the number of people living below the federal poverty level from 44 million to 28 million. While these provisions are not directed at healthcare, they improve the social determinants of health, the conditions in the places where people live, learn, work, and play that affect a wide range of health and quality-of life-risks and outcomes.

In a related development, President Biden extended a special enrollment period to allow people to sign up for health insurance through the federal health insurance marketplace through August 15th. More than three million Americans did so. The extended open enrollment period will allow Americans to take advantage of new savings under ARPA. However, the ARPA subsidy provisions are temporary, lasting for two years, retroactive to January 1, 2021.

In his address to the nation that day, President Biden set a goal of July 4th to mark *"independence from the virus."* To get there, the administration directed states, tribes and territories to make all American adults eligible for the vaccines by May 1st . Biden also was sharply critical of the prior administration's response noting that the country a year ago was *"hit with a virus that was met with silence"* and *"denial."* He also pointed out that the country didn't have nearly enough vaccines when he took office, but soon will with the purchase of hundreds of millions of the three vaccines currently in use.

With ample vaccine supplies, the U.S. began a vaccine vs. virus variants race to recovery. Even with the dawn of the Delta variant in late spring, America's progress in bringing the pandemic under control has been steady. By August 31st , the U.S. had climbed to 26th out of the 37 OECD member nations with a per capita fatality rate of 193.2/100,000 compared with the OECD average of 147.0/100,000. Germany is now 15th of 37 with a per capita fatality rate of 110.1/100,000, France was 24th at 175.1, and the U.K. 28th at 195.7. Canada, our neighbor to the North, fared even better, ranking 10th in the OECD with a per capita fatality rate of 71.5/100,000 (see chart, Chapter 3).

Unfortunately, progress at the state level was distinctly mixed. Concerned about the low vaccination rates and increasing infections in many states, on July 19 CDC Director Dr. Rochelle Walensky warned that the outbreak in the U.S. is becoming a "*pandemic of the unvaccinated*" that continues to hobble America's efforts to put the worst of the Covid-19 pandemic in the rear-view mirror. She noted that nearly all current hospitalizations and deaths are among those who have not been immunized.

In late August, hospitals in six states are virtually out of ICU beds (Alabama, Florida, Georgia, Kentucky, Mississippi and Texas) and four others are close behind (Arkansas, Louisiana, Missouri and Oklahoma). New confirmed cases are averaging more than 150,000/day – ten times what they were in June, and 18% of the new cases are in children. Emergency Rooms in those states are so overloaded with Covid-19 patients that heart attack, stroke and accident victims often are not seen in a timely manner. Worse still, front line clinicians are worn down from 18 months of crisis care – in some instances, there are beds available, but no nurses available to staff them.

One way of assessing the effectiveness of state leadership is to look at the change in fatality rates since mid-year 2020, after the initial Covid-19 surge. The chart below compares the performance of Florida, Georgia and Texas with five states that were hit early in the pandemic (Connecticut, Massachusetts, New Jersey, New York and Washington).

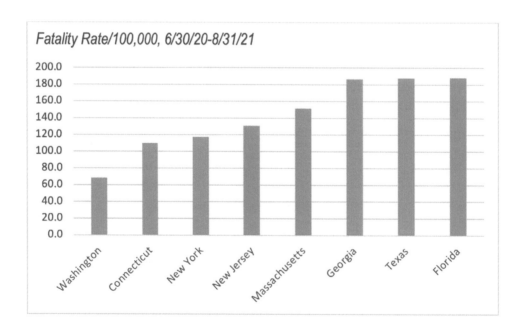

Clearly, the four states to the left did a better job of managing their pandemic response during that 14-month period than did the four states on the right. Whatever the ultimate truth, it's clear that the Trump Administration's failure to take the pandemic seriously resulted in well over 150,000 avoidable American deaths:

- If the U.S. had merely matched the OECD's average fatality rate/100,000 of 147.0, 157,000 more Americans would be alive today.
- If the U.S. had matched Germany's performance (110.1/100,000), 275,000 more Americans would be alive today.
- If the U.S. had matched Canada (71.5/100,000), 373,000 more Americans would be alive today.

Sadly, the U.S. death toll likely will surpass the 675,000 lives lost during the 2018-19 pandemic before September month end. Having failed to apply the lessons learned from history, the U.S. was doomed to repeat it.

Pandemic U. S. 2021 Three Minute Reads

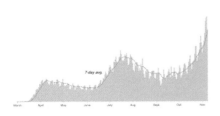

As cases rise, states say they'll work with Biden on virus, Associated Press, 11/9/20

TMR Topline™ - President-Elect Joe Biden announced his coronavirus task force and has begun reaching out to governors to build consensus for a cohesive national strategy to contain the Covid-19 pandemic. New Mexico's Gov. Michelle Lujan Grisham, an early adopter of aggressive pandemic restrictions, praised Biden for "*leading with science and de-politicizing the federal government's pandemic response.*" Idaho Gov. Brad Little wrote an opinion piece Monday imploring people to wear masks, though he said he does not have the authority to issue a statewide mandate. Utah Gov. Gary Herbert ordered a statewide mask mandate and is pausing extracurricular school activities, along with most sports and social gatherings with people outside the household.

Dr. Georges Benjamin, executive director of the American Public Health Association, said "*Part of the problem with the response so far is that there really hasn't been a testing plan, and a contract tracing plan and any kind of meaningful disease containment plan that all of us understood.*" For example, early in the pandemic, President Trump told states that they were responsible for buying their own protective gear and they began bidding against each other for PPE. Biden is asking governors and local leaders to require mask use in public and to normalize social distancing.

TMR's Take –President-Elect Biden intends to replace the scattershot approach to combatting the virus over the last ten months with a plan based on science that crosses party lines and meets the public health challenges of Covid-19.

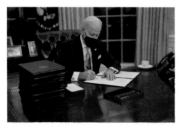

Biden looks to galvanize COVID-19 fight, vaccinations as he takes office, by Susan Heavey, Patricia Zengerle, Reuters, 1/20/21

TMR Topline™ - Inaugurated the day after America's death toll surpassed 400,000, President Biden asked for a moment of silent prayer during his address, stating: *"We're entering what may be the toughest and deadliest period of the virus and must set aside politics and finally face this pandemic as one nation."* Biden's first three Executive Orders targeted Covid-19: requiring masks on federal property, rejoining the World Health Organization and establishing a White House Covid-19 response team led by Jeff Zients. Biden's executive actions are also intended to set an example for state and local officials as they try to rein in the virus and drew praise from U.S. Chamber of Commerce President Suzanne Clark calling it *"a smart and practical approach."*

Biden signs burst of virus orders, vows 'Help is on the way',
by Ricardo Alonso-Zaldivar and Zeke Miller, Associated Press, 1/21/21

TMR Topline™ - The 10 orders signed by Biden are aimed at jump starting his national Covid-19 strategy to increase vaccinations and testing, lay the groundwork for reopening schools and businesses, and immediately increase the use of masks — including a requirement that Americans mask up for travel. Promising stringent adherence to public health guidance, Biden declared: *"To a nation waiting for action, let me be clear on this point: help is on the way."*

Hampered by a lack of cooperation during the transition, Biden's advisors say they don't have a complete understanding of their predecessors' actions on vaccine distribution. When a reporter suggested that his goal of 100 million shots in his first 100 days in office is too low, Biden responded *""When I announced it, you all said it's not possible. Come on, give me a break, man."* Dr. Fauci told reporters that if the vaccination campaign goes well, the U.S. could return to *"a degree of normality"* by the fall.

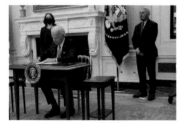

Here's What's in Biden's Executive Orders Aimed at Curbing the Pandemic, by Noah Weiland, New York Times, 1/22/21

TMR Topline™ - The series of Executive orders and presidential directives issued during President Biden's first full day in office signal a more centralized federal response to the spread of Covid-19, including:

- Ramp up the pace of manufacturing and testing.
- Require mask wearing during interstate travel.
- Establish a Pandemic Testing Board.
- Publish guidance for schools and workers.
- Find more treatments for Covid-19 and future pandemics.

Agencies also are directed to identify areas where the administration could invoke the Defense Production Act to increase manufacturing, such as PPE, swabs, reagents, pipettes and syringes.

TMR's Take –Delivering on his campaign promise, President Biden launched an all-out war against the coronavirus that, in less than a year, has claimed more American lives than perished during the four years of World War 2. Had the U.S. merely matched Canada or Germany's performance during 2020, more than 200,000 of our fellow Americans would be alive today. Such leadership is a welcome change from the laissez-faire malign neglect of the prior administration.

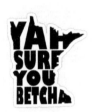

The U.S. Needs More Covid Testing, and Minnesota Has Found a Way, by Susan Berfield and Michelle Fay Cortez, Bloomberg, 1/11/21.

TMR Topline™ - With a progressive governor and a budget surplus, Minnesota has spent $150 million on testing, including a major ramp-up of the saliva test developed at Rutgers last spring. Infinity BiologiX's Oakdale lab, located about 10 miles from downtown St. Paul next to a UPS depot, receives four deliveries daily and processes up to 30,000 tests per day with results available within 48 hours.

The saliva tests are as sensitive and accurate as the nasal PCR tests according to data posted by the FDA and can be self-administered. Governor Walz notes that when neighboring North Dakota and South Dakota had the highest positivity rates in the nation, Minnesota was ranked 21st. *"Our strategy was effective,"* he says. *"but its effectiveness was blunted by the sheer magnitude of cases."*

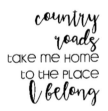

'Little old West Virginia' sets pace on vaccine rollout, by Cuneyt Dil, Associated Press, 1/19/21.

TMR Topline™ - West Virginia rejected the federal partnership with CVS and Walgreens, instead relying on its mom-and-pop pharmacies to vaccinate residents. It was first in the nation to finish offering first doses to nursing home residents by the end of December. Also, 250 local pharmacists set up clinics in rural communities and the Mountaineer state leads the U.S. in per capita vaccination rates.

The initiative has not been error free: one county health department has been barred from the program after administering an antibody treatment to 44 people instead of the vaccine. Noting concerns about vaccine safety, Michael Rotholz of the American Pharmacists Association said: "*having access to a health care provider like a community pharmacist provides a comfort level to the patients and communities.*"

TMR's Take - Kudos to the governors of Minnesota (a Democrat) and West Virginia (a Republican) for their leadership in protecting their residents from Covid-19.

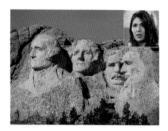

S.D. Governor Gives State High Marks in Handling the Pandemic. Are They Deserved?, by Carmen Heredia Rodriguez, Kaiser Health News/Politifact, 2/12/21

TMR Topline™ - South Dakota Governor Kristi Noem claims that, despite her refusal to enact a mask mandate or close any businesses, her state *"got through it better than virtually every other state."* Asked the reasons for the claim, communications director Ian Fury cited vaccine distribution, unemployment, the number of people moving to the state and the state's $19 million budget surplus. However, its per capita death rate of 201/100,000 at 1/31 places it in the top 10 states, and there were reports in December of Covid patients being transferred out-of-state due to limited ICU capacity. The state experienced less of an economic decline than initially projected due to federal aid and conservative revenue projections. South Dakota is one of the top states in per capita vaccination rates. The article concluded that Noem's statement *"cherry-picked the data, emphasizing the state's economy while giving less weight to the lives lost and the burden of disease its residents suffered."*

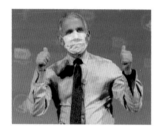

Fauci is awarded a $1 million prize in Israel, including for 'speaking truth to power.', by Isabel Kershner, New York Times, 2/15/21

TMR Topline™ - The three 2020 awards from the Dan David Foundation and Tel Aviv University are for outstanding contributions in public health, noting that *"He has been widely praised for his courage in speaking truth to power in a highly charged environment."* Dr. Anthony Fauci won in the "Present" category for his scientific contributions, including his research and his efforts to inform the public about the pandemic.

TMR's Take - Governor Noem's chutzpah ranks with Belgium's Health Minister Maggie De Block who, despite having the highest fatality rate in the OECD, defended her government's response, noting with pride that Belgium never ran out of hospital beds. August's 10 day Sturgis SD Motorcycle Rally was a super spreader on steroids. Neighboring states might take issue with the governor's claim. Conversely, Israel's recognition of Dr. Fauci is well-deserved.

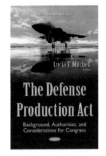

Biden Says He Invoked Production Law For More Vaccine Doses, by Justin Sink, Josh Wingrove and Jennifer Epstein, Bloomberg, 2/16/21

TMR Topline™ - President Joe Biden said that Moderna Inc. and Pfizer Inc. agreed to sell more doses of their coronavirus vaccine to the U.S. faster than planned after he invoked the Defense Production Act, a law that allows the government to nationalize commercial production in emergencies. In a CNN town hall event in Milwaukee on Tuesday, he touted his administration's ramp-up of vaccine shipments while also warning that the pandemic won't soon end: *"We got them to move up time because we used the National Defense Act to be able to help the manufacturing piece of it, to get more equipment."*.

TMR's Take - President Biden's campaign promised that controlling the pandemic was a top priority and his actions since taking office are delivering on that promise.

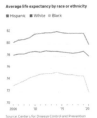

COVID-19 has already cut U.S. life expectancy by a year. For Black Americans, it's worse, PBS News Hour, 2/18/21

TMR Topline™ - A report released by the National Center for Health Statistics, part of the CDC, for the first six months of 2020 show an alarming decline of one year in life expectancy for Americans. Demographer Elizabeth Arias, the report's lead author, noted that Black men are experiencing a drop in life expectancy comparable to 1942-43, when the average American's lifespan dropped by 2.9 years. The 1918-19 pandemic saw U.S. life expectancy drop by 11 years. The U.S. also saw a decline from 2015-17 due to an increase in drug abuse deaths and suicide rates.

TMR's Take - The shocking decline in life expectancy is likely to be higher when data are compiled for the full year since Covid-19 deaths were 100,000 higher during the second half of 2020.

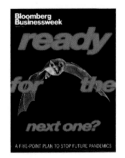

The Five Things to Get Right Before the Next Pandemic, by Robert Langerth, Bloomberg Business Week, 2/3/21

TMR Topline™ - In January 2017, GlaxoSmithKline submitted a 112-page proposal to HHS's Biomedical Advanced Research and Development Authority (BARDA) to prevent future pandemics. Created in 2006, BARDA is charged with developing and procuring drugs and vaccines and ensuring that the U.S. is researching pandemic influenza and other emerging infectious threats. After the 2014 Ebola outbreak, Glaxo researchers wanted to identify viruses likely to cause major epidemics and tackle several concurrently. The proposal was not funded, leaving the world without a key weapon when Covid-19 emerged. Protecting the U.S. from the next pandemic will require:

1. *Increasing pathogen surveillance.* The EcoHealth Alliance suggests tracking emerging viruses so that we can intervene before they wreak havoc. A Johns Hopkins epidemiologist suggests a kind of National Weather Service for pandemics that would help predict the course of emerging pathogens.

2. *Repairing and augmenting the WHO.* In January an independent panel convened by the WHO blasted the current epidemic alert system as *"slow, cumbersome, and indecisive."* The Coalition for Epidemic Preparedness Innovations suggests a *"biological NATO"* to defend the world against developing pathogens.

3. *Genetic sequencing.* Frequent, intensive viral sequencing would help answer questions such as how widely a given strain spreads within a community like a school and whether the strain might mutate to become resistant to existing vaccines.

4. *Developing more vaccines, faster.* Strategies include getting to phase 3 clinical trials faster and maintaining standby manufacturing capacity and supplies.

5. *Ironing out distribution and logistics.* Adapting logistics in a healthcare system as large and complicated as the U.S. takes months of advanced planning, and databases to keep track of everything. It didn't happen in 2020.

TMR's Take - The author's right: failing to put more extensive infrastructure in place ahead of time was a blunder that ranks with the May 2018 decision to disband the NSC's pandemic response unit. President Biden's $20 billion proposal to speed up vaccination rollouts is a start, but a complete plan is needed. Covid-19 is the 5th major outbreak of the 21st century. It won't be the last.

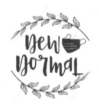

The Most Likely Timeline for Life to Return to Normal, by Joe Pinsker, The Atlantic, 2/24/21

TMR Topline™ - The author expects an uncertain spring, an amazing summer, a cautious fall and winter, and finally, relief. Given that the wild card is the potential emergence of virulent vaccine-resistant variants, daily life will continue to be far from normal for the next few months. By late spring, small gatherings of vaccinated people should be feasible. At some point between June and September, the combination of widespread vaccinations and warmer weather may make many activities much safer, including taking public transit, being in a workplace, dining inside restaurants, and traveling domestically.

However, experts don't foresee the return of indoor concerts, full stadiums or high levels of international travel yet. The summer reprieve could be temporary. Some resurgence of the virus is likely in the fall as activities move indoors. If stubborn variants do circulate, new vaccines should be able to tame them relatively quickly. While there might be a need to revert to some of the precautions from earlier in the pandemic, the disruptions to daily life are likely to be short-lived. Beyond next winter, experts' predict a return to whatever qualifies as normal post-pandemic. The virus will still exist, but like the flu it will circulate primarily in the colder months.

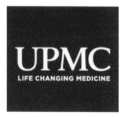

Fighting COVID on three fronts, by Jennifer Lubell, Modern Healthcare, 2/28/21

TMR Topline™ - Western Pennsylvania's largest health system has continuously applied new learnings in its battle against Covid-19. Here are three:

General Masking. UPMC took a closer look at its mask strategy. *"Meaning, how many people had been fit-tested for N-95 masks? How available were they? Did we have the best solutions?"* said UPMC Chief Quality Officer Tami Minnier. UPMC learned their degree of preparedness needed to be a notch higher on an ongoing basis.

Contact tracing. UPMC created a contact tracing app that has allowed the health system to stay ahead on Covid exposures and reduce or prevent outbreaks. Nearly all employee exposures came from community events outside of work. *"Our contact tracing app really allowed us to contain things quickly,"* Minnier said.

Mass vaccination. UPMC had researched ways to accelerate mass vaccinations, testing its approaches with the influenza vaccines. When the pandemic began, the health system had a structure in place to mass vaccinate its employees and workers in nearby health systems. As of mid-February, 80% of UPMC's 90,000 healthcare employees had completed their first dose and most had received their second.

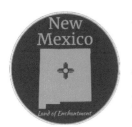

How New Mexico Became the State With the Highest Rate of Full Vaccinations, by Simon Romero, New York Times, 4/14/21

TMR Topline™ - With one of the country's highest poverty rates and lowest hospital beds per capita, New Mexico has produced one of the most efficient vaccine rollouts in the U.S.: 57% of its adult population have received at least one dose of vaccine. Experts attribute the success to a combination of homegrown technological expertise, cooperation between state and local agencies and a focus by elected officials on combating the virus. Gov. Michelle Lujan Grisham, a former state health secretary, set the tone by adopting social distancing measures from the start of the crisis despite some fierce opposition. She mobilized the New Mexico National Guard and Civil Air Patrol to operate a large vaccine distribution center in Albuquerque and staff drive-through testing sites and set up a centralized vaccine portal for all residents to sign up for shots. Native Americans are getting the vaccine at close to the same rate as Anglos in the state. Ms. Lujan Grisham said, *"I fully believe New Mexico can be the first state to reach herd immunity and be the first to begin operating in the new post-pandemic 'normal' the right way, the safe way."*

TMR's Take - Like West Virginia's vaccine rollout (see TMR January 2021-3), solid gubernatorial leadership can make a huge difference in protecting their state's residents from Covid-19.

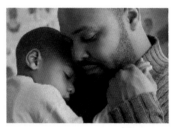

Estimates and Projections of COVID-19 and Parental Death in the US, by Rachel Kidman, Rachel Margolis, Emily Smith-Greenway et. al. JAMA Pediatrics 3/5/21

TMR Topline ™ -The authors developed a model to project the number of children who have lost at least one parent to the Covid-19 pandemic through February 2021 and estimated that 37,300 children up to age 17 had lost at least one parent. Children of color were disproportionately affected. Three-quarters of those who lost parents were adolescents. Children who lose a parent are at higher risk of traumatic grief, depression, poor educational outcomes, and unintentional death or suicide. The sudden loss of a parent to Covid-19 is traumatizing for children and leaves surviving family members ill prepared to deal with the new situation. The pandemic mitigation strategies (social isolation, distance learning, and economic hardship) leave bereaved children without the supports needed to cope with the tragedy.

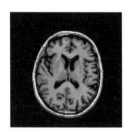

Some Children With Covid-Related Syndrome Develop Neurological Symptoms, by Pam Belluck, New York Times 4/13/21

TMR Topline ™ – Past reports about Multisystem Inflammatory Syndrome in Children (MIS-C) focused on physical symptoms such as rash, abdominal pain, red eyes and heart problems like low blood pressure, shock and difficulty pumping blood. A new study from University College London's Institute of Neurology describes 46 children treated at one London hospital: 24 experienced neurological symptoms including hallucinations, confusion, speech impairments and problems with balance and coordination. Study co-author Dr. Omar Abdel-Mannan said those patients were twice as likely as those without neurological symptoms to need ventilators because they were *"very unwell with systemic shock as part of their hyperinflammatory state."*

A majority of those afflicted were *"nonwhite,"* a pattern that public health experts believe reflects the disproportionate way the pandemic has affected communities of color. Nearly two-thirds were male, and the median age was 10. All 24 had headaches and 14 had confusion, problems with memory or attention. Six experienced hallucinations, including *"describing people in the room that were not there or seeing cartoons or animals moving on the walls,"* Dr. Abdel-Mannan said. Some experienced auditory hallucinations involving *"hearing voices of people not present."* There were no deaths and *"almost all children made a complete functional recovery."* The research team will follow these children to learn if any experience long-term cognitive or psychological effects. MIS-C usually appears 2-6 weeks after a Covid-19 infection, often producing mild or no symptoms. It's rare but can be serious. The CDC reports 3,165 cases including 36 deaths through March 2021.

TMR's Take - While most think of Covid-19 as an adult disease, both articles highlight the full range of emotional and physical difficulties that children can experience due to the pandemic.

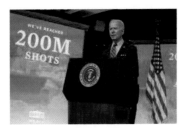

Biden Says Goal Of 200 Million COVID-19 Vaccinations In 100 Days Has Been Met, by Brian Naylor, NPR, 4/21/21

TMR Topline™ - President Biden announced that Americans have received 200 million vaccinations since taking office, double his initial goal of 100 million in his first 100 days. By 4/25, more of half of adult Americans will have had at least one shot, including 80% of those over 65. He also announced the availability of tax credits to employers who give their workers paid leave to get a shot. *"No working American should lose a single dollar from their paycheck because they are doing their patriotic duty to get vaccinated,"* Biden said. As of 4/19, all Americans 16 and older are eligible to get vaccinated.

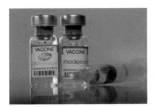

As more data shows COVID-19 vaccines highly effective in teens, numbers could reverse a 'lag phase' on inoculations, by John Bacon, USA Today, 5/6/21

TMR Topline™ - Moderna has reported that its vaccine is showing a 96% effectiveness rate in Phase 2/3 testing of adolescents ages 12 to 17. The vaccine was generally well tolerated, and most adverse events were mild or moderate in severity. Pfizer has reported its Covid-19 vaccine was 100% effective in a study of adolescents ages 12 to 15. Emergency use authorization for its vaccine is expected soon. These positive results come at a time when the rate of daily vaccinations has declined due in part to the pause in J&J's one-shot vaccine due to concerns about blood clots. The data could help curb broader vaccine hesitancy, which has been partly to blame for a slowdown in daily shots. Translating the good news into increased vaccination rates will require effective public health messaging.

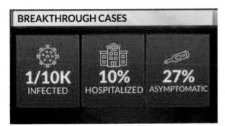

'Breakthrough' infections are rare, and just 2% result in COVID-19 deaths, CDC says, by Melissa Healy, Los Angeles Times, 5/26/21

TMR Topline™ - During a four-month span when more than 100 million Americans were vaccinated, 10,262 post-vaccination infections were reported and 160 – all between the age of 71 and 89 – died, less than 2% of those with *"breakthrough"* infections. Asked about the vaccines, Vanderbilt University epidemiologist Dr. William Schaffner stated: *"It gives them an A, if not an A-plus. It shows that infections among vaccinated people are, first of all, unusual. And second, that there are very few among these infections that are linked to deaths."* Even when breakthrough infections occurred, the vaccines likely prevented severe disease, hospitalizations and deaths in those who got them. The study also found that variants were not more likely to cause breakthrough infections. Dr. Schaffner concluded: *"The vaccines are working,"* adding that we have *"to see how long vaccines' protection lasts. And we have to keep monitoring for those variants. We must remain on alert."*

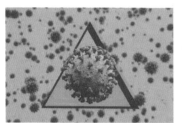

US surgeon general warns unvaccinated people are at risk from a potentially more dangerous Covid-19 variant, by Travis Caldwell, CNN, 6/10/21

TMR Topline™ - U.S. Surgeon-General Dr. Vivek Murthy has issued a warning: *"For those who are unvaccinated, they are increasingly at risk as more and more variants develop,"* specifically citing the B.1.617.2, or Delta variant, first identified in India. *"The news about the Delta variant is evidence of really why it's so important for us to get vaccinated as soon as possible,"* he said, adding that the variant is more transmissible and potentially more dangerous. The Delta variant now is the dominant variant in the U.K. and accounts for more than 6% of sequenced virus in the U.S. According to the CDC, Connecticut, Maine, Maryland, Massachusetts, New Hampshire, New Jersey, Rhode Island and Vermont have vaccinated more than 50% of their population while Alabama, Arkansas, Louisiana, Mississippi, Tennessee and Wyoming have among the lowest vaccination rates in the country. A U.K. study found that the Pfizer vaccine was highly effective against the Delta variant after two doses.

TMR's Take - Heed Dr. Murthy's lifesaving advice!

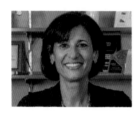

Nearly all COVID deaths in US are now among unvaccinated, by Carla K. Johnson and Mike Stobbe, Associated Press, 6/24/21

TMR Topline™ - AP's analysis of available government data from May shows that *"breakthrough"* infections in fully vaccinated people accounted for fewer than 1,200 of more than 853,000 Covid-19 hospitalizations (0.14%). About 150 of May's more than 18,000 Covid-19 deaths were in fully vaccinated people. Deaths in the U.S. have plummeted from a peak of more than 3,400/day on average in mid-January, to less than 300/day now. CDC Director Dr. Rochelle Walensky said during Tuesday's White House coronavirus briefing that the vaccine is so effective that *"nearly every death, especially among adults, due to Covid-19, is, at this point, entirely preventable."* She called such deaths *"particularly tragic."* Experts predict that preventable deaths will continue with unvaccinated pockets of the nation having outbreaks next fall and winter. The University of Washington's modeling suggests the U.S. will hit 1,000 deaths per day next year.

TMR Take's – Heed the doctors lifesaving advice! If you haven't already done so, **_get vaccinated!_** The life you save may be your own

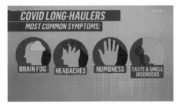

CDC's new guidance for treating COVID-19 long-haulers warns against relying on labs, imaging results alone, by Dave Muoio, Fierce Healthcare, 6/17/21

TMR Topline™ - The CDC released interim guidance for healthcare providers treating patients with post-Covid conditions. Often referred to as *"long Covid,"* these are a wide range of physical and mental health issues that sometimes persist four or more weeks after a Covid-19 infection. These include heart palpitations, cognitive impairment, insomnia, diarrhea and post-exertional malaise, a worsening of symptoms following physical or mental exertion. According to the CDC, many patients' post-Covid conditions can be managed by primary care providers. A study by FAIR Health found that more than 23% of patients who had Covid-19 experienced one or more post-Covid conditions 30 days after their initial diagnosis. Pain, breathing difficulties, hyperlipidemia, malaise and fatigue and hypertension were the five most common post-Covid conditions, and were more common among females than males. The study also found a higher risk of mortality after acute treatment.

TMR's Take - For nearly one of four Covid survivors, beating the infection is not the end of the battle. For some, the symptoms continue to persist and may last for years. Preventing the next pandemic should be the #1 priority on America's public health agenda.

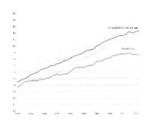

The Pandemic Led To The Biggest Drop In U.S. Life Expectancy Since WWII, Study Finds, by Allison Aubrey, NPR, 6/23/21

TMR Topline™ - According to a new study published in the British Medical Journal, life expectancy in the U.S. has declined from 78.9 years in 2014 to 76.9 years at 2020-year end. African Americans and Hispanic Americans were especially hard hit with declines of 3.3 and 3.9 years, respectively. Study author Stephen Woolf of the Virginia Commonwealth University School of Medicine stated: *"We have not seen a decrease like this since World War II. It's a horrific decrease in life expectancy,"* further noting that disruptions in behavioral health and chronic disease management contributed to the decline. Lesley Curtis, chair of the Department of Population Health Sciences at Duke University School of Medicine said, *"It is impossible to look at these findings and not see a reflection of the systemic racism in the U.S."* Dr. Richard Besser, president of the Robert Wood Johnson Foundation said *"This study further destroys the myth that the United States is the healthiest place in the world to live. For example, life expectancy in Princeton, NJ—a predominantly White community—is 14 years higher than Trenton, NJ, a predominantly Black and Latino city only 14 miles away."*

The U.S. has been losing ground compared with other wealthy countries, said Magali Barbieri of the University of California, Berkeley, in an editorial published alongside the new study. The decline in life expectancy was only 0.22 years in a peer group of 16 high income countries. Woolf concluded *"The U.S. has some of the best hospitals and some of the greatest scientists. But other countries do far better in getting quality medical care to their population. We have big gaps in getting care to people who need it most, when they need it most."*

TMR's Take - For vaccinated Americans, the Covid-19 pandemic appears under control, but what a toll it has taken, especially among communities of color. At 12/31/20, 343,818 Americans had perished; more than 260,000 have died since then so U.S. life expectancy will continue to plummet. Your Editor has often stated that America has the most thoroughly trained physicians and best-equipped hospitals in the world but does not deliver health to its population.

Deaths and Hospitalizations Averted by Rapid U.S. Vaccination Rollout, by Alison Galvani, Seyed M. Moghadas and Eric C. Schneider, The Commonwealth Fund, Issue Briefs, 7/7/21

TMR Topline™ - By 7/2, the U.S. had administered more than 328 million vaccine doses, with 67% of adults having received at least one dose. The authors modeled the impact of the vaccination program (see How We Conducted This Study). The vaccination campaign markedly curbed the U.S. pandemic. Without it, there would have been about 279,000 more deaths and up to 1.25 million more hospitalizations by 6/30 (see chart).

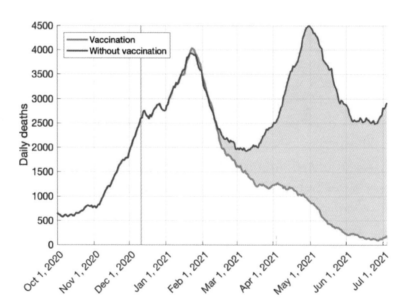

If the U.S. had vaccinated at half the pace, there would have been about 121,000 additional deaths. They concluded: *"Our results demonstrate the extraordinary impact of rapidly vaccinating a large share of the population to prevent hospitalizations and deaths. The speed of vaccination seems to have prevented another potential wave of the U.S. pandemic in April that might otherwise have been triggered by the Alpha and Gamma variants."*

TMR Take – Had the Biden Administration continued vaccinating at the same rate as its predecessor, roughly 200,000 more Americans would have perished by 6/30.

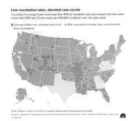

Hospitals in low-vaccination states struggle as COVID-19 surges, by Steven Ross Johnson, Modern Healthcare, 7/13/21

TMR Topline™ - States with the highest seven-day average increases in cases also have some of the country's lowest vaccination rates. CoxHealth is one of the health systems at the forefront. Serving patients in southwestern Missouri and northwestern Arkansas, it has gone from having about 20 patients a day hospitalized for Covid-19 related illnesses in May to more than 100 by July. In Springfield Missouri, the number of Covid-19 related inpatients jumped from 76 on June 8 to 192 by July 8.

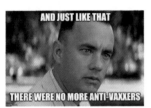

COVID-19 'is becoming a pandemic of the unvaccinated,' CDC director says, by Heather Hollingsworth and Josh Funk, Associated Press, 7/16/21

TMR Topline™ - The Covid-19 comeback is putting pressure on hospitals at a time when some are busy just trying to catch up on elective procedures that were postponed during the pandemic. Staff members are worn out and finding traveling nurses to boost their ranks can be tough. *"I really think of it as a war and how long can you stay on the front line,"* said Dr. Mark Rosenberg, president of the American College of Emergency Physicians. *"And how many times do you want to go back for another tour of duty. Eventually you just don't want to do it."* The fear now is that hospitals might have to postpone non-Covid-19-related care again — and risk the potential health consequences for patients. CDC Director Dr. Rochelle Walensky warned that the outbreak in the U.S. is becoming *"a pandemic of the unvaccinated"* because nearly all hospital admissions and deaths are among those who hadn't been immunized.

TMR's Take - Dr. Walensky's right! If you haven't done so, *get vaccinated!* The life you save may be your own.

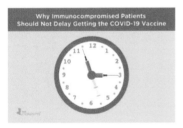

U.S. plans to give extra COVID-19 shots to at-risk Americans, Fauci says, by Trevor Hunnicutt, Carl O'Donnell Reuters, 8/5/21

TMR Topline™ - The CDC is working to make third doses available sooner to immunocompromised people who may not be sufficiently protected by their existing Covid-19 vaccinations. *"It is extremely important for us to move to get those individuals their boosters and we are now working on that,"* Fauci said. The U.S. is joining Germany, France and Israel in giving booster shots, given rising cases resulting from the spread of the contagious Delta variant.

TMR's Take –Why not provide booster shots to the 7 million immunocompromised Americans **and** honor the WHO's moratorium request? While Moderna and Pfizer both are urging booster shots after 6 months, data shows their vaccines retain a high degree of effectiveness. By September month-end more data will be available to decide whether booster shots are needed.

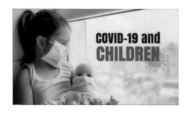

COVID-19 cases in children surge 84% in 1 week, study finds, by Patrick Reilly, New York Post, 8/5/21

TMR Topline™ - the American Academy of Pediatrics [AAP] teamed up with Children's Hospitals of America to help collect and share data on pediatric Covid-19 cases. They were 14.3% of cumulative cases; that share rose to 19% for the week ended 7/29. While severe illness due to Covid-19 is uncommon among children, AAP is concerned about the millions of children returning to school over the next month and expressed an *"urgent need"* to learn more about the pandemic's long-term effects on children's physical, mental and emotional health. According to the CDC, 526 children have died from the virus; 4.2 million children have tested positive for the virus.

TMR's Take - Currently, 1,600 children are hospitalized with Covid-19. Florida Gov. Ron DeSantis has made it illegal for school boards to mandate mask requirements in schools, and the state has the 3rd highest per capita rate of Covid-19 infections in the world behind Louisiana and Botswana. Gov. Greg Abbott's Texas is not far behind, also banning mask mandates. Last century, the comedy duo of Abbott & Costello was frightfully funny; today, the gubernatorial duo of Abbott & DeSantis is just frightening.

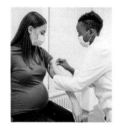

CDC urges COVID vaccines during pregnancy as delta surges, by Lindsey Tanner and Mike Stobbe, Associated Press, 8/11/21

TMR Topline™ - The CDC is urging all pregnant women to get the Covid-19 vaccine as hospitals are seeing disturbing numbers of unvaccinated mothers-to-be seriously ill with the virus. About 23% have received at least one dose of vaccine. A CDC analysis of safety data on 2,500 women showed no increased risks of miscarriage for those who received at least one dose of the vaccine before 20 weeks of pregnancy. Pregnancy-related changes in body functions may explain why the virus can be dangerous for mothers-to-be. These include reduced lung capacity and adjustments in the disease-fighting immune system that protect and help the fetus grow. The new advice also applies to nursing mothers and women planning to get pregnant.

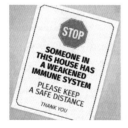

CDC Recommends 3rd Vaccine Dose For Immunocompromised People, by Joe Neel, NPR, 8/13/21

TMR Topline™ - Following FDA approval, the CDC is recommending a third shot of the Pfizer or Moderna vaccine for immunocompromised people (2.7% of U.S. adults, about 7 million). One U.S. study shows 40- 44% of hospitalized breakthrough cases are in immuno-compromised people. People with the following conditions should take a third dose:

- Been receiving active cancer treatment for tumors or cancers of the blood.
- Received an organ transplant and are taking medicine to suppress the immune system.

- Received a stem cell transplant within the last two years or are taking medicine to suppress the immune system.
- Moderate or severe primary immunodeficiency.
- Advanced or untreated HIV infection.
- Active treatment with high-dose corticosteroids or other drugs that may suppress your immune response.

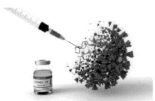

Get Vaccinated Even If You've Gotten COVID-19, Study Suggests, by Frank Diamond and Kevin Kavanaugh, MD, Infection Control Today, 8/13/21

TMR Topline™ - A recent study in the CDC's *Morbidity and Mortality Weekly Report* examined data from Kentucky residents who were infected with Covid-19 in 2020, then identified those reinfected in May and June 2021. Unvaccinated residents with natural immunity were 2.3 times more likely to have breakthrough infections than those Covid-19 survivors who were vaccinated.

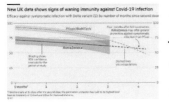

New data shows waning COVID-19 vaccine efficacy, building case for boosters, by Lisa M. Krieger, Bay Area News Group, 8/18/21

TMR Topline™ - Three new studies released by the CDC show that protection from infection has been waning since earlier this year. In one study, the decline was modest, dropping from 92% to 80%. In the second, it was more dramatic, falling from 75% to 53%. A third study found that protection fell from 76% to 42% among recipients of the Pfizer vaccine and from 86% to 76% among recipients of the Moderna vaccine. These findings are spurring the campaign to boost Americans' immunity by administering a third dose of the vaccine. *"You don't want to find yourself behind, playing catch up,"* said NIAID Director Dr. Anthony S. Fauci, noting that a *"booster"* vaccine can trigger a sudden, ten-fold jump in antibody levels. Pending consent from the FDA and the CDC, boosters will be available starting the week of September 20th.

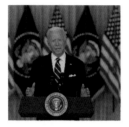

Biden says some Americans will be eligible for booster shots in September. by Sharon LaFraniere and Apoorva Mandavilli, New York Times, 8/18/21

TMR Topline™ - President Biden announced several steps being taken to combat the spread of Covid-19's delta variant including strongly recommending booster shots for vaccinated Americans, directing the Education Secretary to *"use all of his authority, and legal action if appropriate,"* to deter states from banning universal masking in classrooms, and making employee vaccination a condition for nursing homes to receive Medicare and Medicaid funding. Senior federal officials said that the booster strategy stemmed from new data showing that vaccine efficacy against infection and mild disease wanes over time.

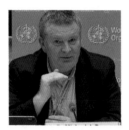

As U.S. promotes booster shots against Covid, moral questions arise over vaccine equity, by Erik Ortiz, NBC News, 8/18/21

TMR Topline™ - The announcement that Covid-19 booster shots will be available to all Americans next month triggered an immediate response from Dr. Michael Ryan, emergencies chief at the WHO: *"We're planning to hand out extra life jackets to people who already have life jackets, while we're leaving other people to drown without a single life jacket."* CDC Director Dr. Rochelle Walensky addressed the criticism: *"I don't think this is a choice in terms of if we have to choose one or the other. We're going to do both and we have been doing both,"* noting that the U.S. anticipates giving 100 million booster shots by the end of the year, while distributing 200 million vaccines worldwide.

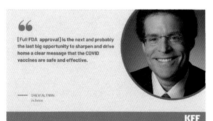

How Full FDA Approval Could Spur Vaccination, by Drew Altman, Axios, 8/13/21

TMR Topline™ - KFF President and CEO Drew Altman is widely respected as a leading expert on health policy issues – and has New Jersey roots. Early in his career, he served as Commissioner of the Department of Human Services and VP at the Robert Wood Johnson Foundation. Data from KFF Vaccine Monitor surveys indicate that 31% of the unvaccinated would be more likely to get vaccinated if the FDA moved vaccines from an EUA to full approval. More than half are unsure what the status of FDA approval is. Approval also offers an opportunity to clear up substantial public confusion.

Bottom line: It's the next, and probably the last,big opportunity to sharpen and drive home a clear message that the Covid vaccines are safe and effective.

TMR Take – Altman's right! America's war against the *"pandemic of the unvaccinated"* is beginning to feel like a 21st century equivalent of the Civil War. Its mission – eliminate an outrageously contagious and deadly virus. It's appalling that many states now look like Queens did in April 2020 when New York Metro was the epicenter of the global pandemic. Mississippi, Louisiana, Arizona, Alabama and South Dakota now have per capita fatality rates comparable to the northeastern states that were hit hard early. Did they learn nothing or did their leaders choose to ignore the science?

A recent Commonwealth Fund study shows that Florida and Texas could have averted 4,700 deaths by the end of July if their vaccination coverage was comparable to the five highest-performing states (Vermont, Connecticut, Massachusetts, Maine, and Rhode Island with 74% of adults fully vaccinated). In his newsletter, Dr. Sanjay Gupta cited a study that found that other mitigation measures – such as physical distancing and handwashing – are *"insufficient by themselves"* in curbing the pandemic without mask use, too. Yet, Governors Abbott and DeSantis have banned masks in schools. Last century, the comedic duo of Abbott & Costello was frightfully funny; today, the gubernatorial duo of Abbott & DeSantis is just frightening. In the ultimate irony, Fox News has mandated that its employees must upload their vaccine status into an internal database. So, ignore their anchors, heed your physician and ***GET VACCINATED!***

CHAPTER 5

Provider Stress, Turnover and Burnout Skyrocket

THE 2011 PASSAGE OF THE AFFORDABLE CARE ACT PROVED TO BE BOTH A BLESSING AND A CURSE FOR healthcare providers. By expanding access to care for previously uninsured Americans, demand for services surged, further stressing frontline clinicians. Hospital systems grew rapidly through vertical and horizontal acquisitions to build critical mass and secure a competitive advantage in negotiating managed care contracts. Still, 60% of hospitals were barely breaking even or operating at a loss, and rural hospitals were closing at a rate of two per month. The increased complexities of dealing with insurers prior authorization requirements and implementing electronic health records (EHRs) drove thousands of small practices to merge with health systems or larger physician groups.

Prior to the pandemic, one study reported that 42% of physicians had experienced burnout at some point in their careers, the highest percentage of any profession. The American Association of Medical Colleges reports annually on the projected future physician shortage. Its latest projection of physician shortages by 2025 is 40% higher than the 2017 projection.

While France has had full interoperability since 1998 and Germany since 2008, America's freewheeling approach has produced systems that often turn physicians and nurses into highly skilled data entry clerks. When data is shared between different EHR systems, error rates of up to 18% occur. Rather than facilitating patient care and improving outcomes, EHRs have become a significant contributor to clinician burnout.

And then, Covid-19 entered the scene and hard-hit areas had to respond on the fly.

Americans watching the evening news were treated to scenes of overwhelmed Metro New York area hospitals with nurses using trash bags as protective gear due to rampant shortages of personal protective equipment (PPE) as well as mobile morgues and refrigerated trucks outside many hospitals - even a shortage of body bags. ICU nurses and cell phones became the sole link to their families for dying patients. As Covid-19 admissions surged, hospitals had to reduce or eliminate elective procedures. Fortunately, the use of telemedicine rapidly expanded to maintain non-Covid-19 patient care where possible. Sadly, more than 3,600 hospital workers have died from Covid-19.

With the best-equipped hospitals and most thoroughly trained physicians in the world, America excels at diagnosing, treating and curing illnesses. Covid-19 clearly stress-tested that combination of skills when it struck Metro New York in March 2020. In America's most densely populated state, New Jersey hospitals worked collaboratively with each other and state officials to develop models and methodologies to guide a data-driven and formulaic approach to sharing and utilizing information to beat back the virus. Learning on the fly, Chief Medical Officers and Chief Nursing Officers held daily teleconferences to share success and failures, what treatments and protocols worked well and what should be set aside. It worked. In April 2020, a patient hospitalized with Covid-19 had a 26.7% likelihood of death. By February 2021, that had dropped to 11.4%.

Similarly, the case fatality rate (# of deaths/# of cases x 100) was 8.2% at April 30, 2020. That percentage might be slightly overstated as testing was not widely prevalent then. By year end, it had declined to 2.2% and has continued to decline. At August 30, 2021, it was 1.9%, a 13.6% improvement over 2020-year end.

Many doctors and nurses have left or are considering leaving the profession, because they report suffering from exhaustion, stress, burnout and PTSD from the constant and never-ending pressure to treat highly contagious patients. In March 2021 alone, 1.5 million women left their jobs in healthcare. In a recent survey 15% of physicians under the age of 45 have said that they plan to retire based on the current stress level of practicing medicine. Turnover in nursing homes is now more than 100% for nurses and certified nursing aides.

Sadly, about 80 million vaccine-eligible Americans have refused to comply with the CDC's public health guidelines, especially in the southeast. Although the vaccines have proven to be safe and effective and the Pfizer-BioNTech vaccine has received full approval from the FDA, millions have refused to take them, then show up in emergency rooms infected with Covid-19 and pleading for the vaccine.

With the Delta variant raging and the Mu variant emerging, hospitals in states with low adult vaccination rates are at or near ICU capacity. Severe staffing shortages see traveling nurses, when available, commanding exorbitant fees to treat the *"pandemic of the unvaccinated."*

The 31 articles summarized in this chapter cover the following topics, including:

- Telehealth's success during the pandemic and its continuing viability.
- The challenging future of post-pandemic healthcare.
- The pandemic's impact on the practice of medicine.
- Clinician burnout – who will be left to provide care?
- Will hospital volumes ever return to pre-pandemic levels?

Provider Issues Three Minute Reads

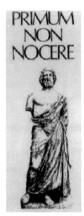

Healthcare leaders fear COVID-19's impact once the storm has passed, by Dr. Halee Fischer-Wright, CEO, Medical Group Management Association, Modern Healthcare,

TMR Topline™ - In a compelling commentary, Dr. Wright laid out critical post-pandemic concerns of America's physician practices, hospitals and health systems following a survey of MGMA's governing affairs council. Noting that the effects of the pandemic are going to be felt long after this storm has passed, Dr. Wright expressed ongoing concern about the lack of personal protective equipment and the risks being faced by physicians, 25% of whom already are in the high-risk category. She expects even further increase in the high stress and burnout rate among physicians, noting that physicians already commit suicide at double the rate of the general population.

Other post-pandemic concerns noted include:

- The need to move to a system based more on preventive care and true public health at a time when providers are psychologically depleted.
- CMS and HHS will use the relief package to accelerate the move to value-based care.
- MGMA's biggest long-term concern is about the financial impact of the crisis, and that the federal government will lower healthcare payments to recoup part of the $2 trillion rescue package.

TMR's Take - We hear Dr. Wright loud and clear. Post-pandemic American healthcare will never be the same.

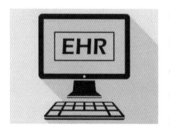

Coronavirus pandemic puts focus on strengths, weaknesses of EHRs, by Nathan Eddy, Healthcare IT News, 3/26/20

TMR Topline™ - The article delves into the key limitations of current EHR architecture: these systems have not been designed to store and share data between disparate and independently functioning systems. As a result, clinicians will have difficulty finding the actionable information they need for decision-making, which in turn will delay patient care.

The article attributes these shortcomings to the fact that U.S. EHR providers are driven by for-profit interests and are highly competitive, but not highly coordinated. HHS released its final interoperability rule 3/9, mandating standards-based exchange of health information through application programming interfaces, or APIs.

TMR's Take - While other OECD countries have achieved full interoperability, the U.S. remains years behind. EHRs that are clunky, inefficient, and not intuitive are a major contributor to physician burnout.

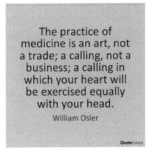

The practice of medicine is an art, not a trade; a calling, not a business; a calling in which your heart will be exercised equally with your head.
William Osler

Will 2020 Be the Year That Medicine Was Saved?, by Drs. Ezekiel J. Emanuel and Amol S. Navathe, NY Times, 4/14/20

TMR Topline™ - The authors describe three major changes that may be Covid-19's silver lining: 1. Telemedicine is now everywhere; 2. Treatment for chronic conditions is moving from doctors seeing patients in hospitals to visiting nurses caring for patients at home; and 3. the use of ineffective or low-value medications, laboratory tests, pre-natal interventions, and diagnostic and surgical procedures has decreased. Unless policies are enacted to preserve them, physicians and hospitals may reverse them. The doctors prescribe three recommendations for medical practices:

1. financially support practices if they stay independent.
2. virtual visits should be reimbursed at the same rate as office visits; and
3. stabilize revenue for all doctors.

They also propose three changes to keep hospitals financially stable without performing unnecessary procedures to generate revenue:

1. Congress should require Medicare to reassess payment for the top 100 elective procedures.
2. hospitals should be required to offer all low-risk patients a care-at-home option; and
3. Medicare payment for any service or procedure should be site neutral.

TMR's Take - The doctors have made an accurate diagnosis. However, their treatment plan will require Sisyphean efforts for enactment.

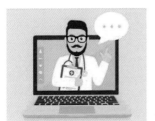

The Transition from Reimagining to Recreating Health Care Is Now, by Judd E. Hollander, MD and Frank D. Sites, MHA, BSN, RN, NEJM Catalyst, 4/8/20

TMR Topline™ - The authors emphasize that telemedicine is a delivery mechanism and dispel five myths delaying its reality:

1. Telemedicine is too hard.
2. Patients prioritize existing relationships with their provider over transactional episodic care.
3. You cannot do a physical examination.
4. Virtual visits are less effective than in-person visits.
5. There is not a payment model supporting telemedicine.

Importantly, the authors chart a practical path to a reality where payers, providers and patients have aligned incentives, and an appreciation that telemedicine is not a new type of medicine, but rather simply a care delivery mechanism that can be utilized with some patients, some of the time, to provide high-quality care.

TMR's Take - While there are regulatory and credentialing issues as remaining "speed bumps," telemedicine as a care delivery mechanism clearly has arrived!

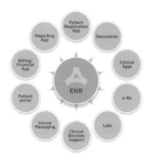

Tips for physician practices: managing the operational, financial challenges of COVID-19 and beyond, by Paola Turchi, Becker's Hospital Review, 5/13/20

TMR Topline™ - MGMA's 4/14 survey found that 97% of medical practices have been adversely affected by the Covid-19 pandemic, averaging more than a 55% decrease in revenue and patient volume. The article describes five federal programs to support medical practices and provides practical advice on coding, accounts receivable management, managing scheduling volumes and preparing for a second wave.

TMR's Take - While it may seem counterintuitive given the public's fear of Covid-19, our hospitals and doctor's offices are safer due to the precautions taken

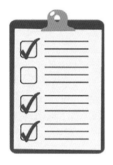

Amid the Coronavirus Crisis, a Regimen for Reentry, by Atul Gawande, MD, The New Yorker, 5/15/20

TMR Topline™ - The author of "The Checklist Manifesto" provides sage advice on reopening the economy. Want to have employees work safely, with each other and with their customers? Emulate the practices at your community hospital. With more than 75,000 employees, Mass General Brigham has minimized workplace transmissions of the Covid-19 virus despite Boston being a pandemic hotspot. How? By implementing hygiene measures, screening, distancing, and masks. Each has flaws. Skip one, and the treatment won't work. But, when taken together, and taken seriously, they shut down the virus.

TMR's Take - While it may seem counterintuitive given the public's fear of Covid-19, our hospitals and doctor's offices are safer due to the precautions taken.

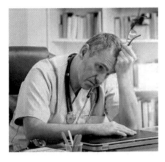

Primary care doctors experience more burnout and anxiety than other healthcare professionals: research, by Heather Landi, Fierce Healthcare, 6/2/20

TMR Topline™ - Conducted by George Mason University's College of Health and Human Services prior to the pandemic and published in the Journal of the American Board of Family Medicine, the survey of 1,243 healthcare professionals from 154 small- and medium-sized Virginia primary care practices found that 31.6% of physicians reported burnout. Physicians who reported increasing anxiety and withdrawal were nearly three times as likely to report burnout. Staff reporting burnout ranged from 17.2-18.9%. Such practices face more challenges adapting to disruptive change including adopting and using electronic health records and compliance with regulatory requirements and payer "speed bumps" such as prior authorization requirements and denials.

TMR's Take - Imagine what the findings might be post-pandemic. At a time when the U.S. shortage of PCPs is growing, so is burnout. It would be interested to see the survey repeated, but also broadened to include PCPs in multispecialty group practices where clinicians have better support so that they can focus on patient care.

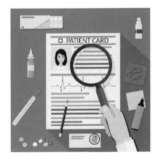

ONC weighs pros and cons of national patient identifier, by Jessica Kim Cohen, Modern Healthcare 6/1/20

TMR Topline™ - HHS' Office of the National Coordinator (ONC) for Health Information Technology convened a panel of 20 experts to discuss the role that a national patient identifier (NPI) could play in improving patient-matching across healthcare organizations. Last year, Congress mandated that the ONC evaluate current patient identification practices and recommend future approaches. Mismatched and unmatched records across various providers can result in waste (duplicative tests) and incorrect clinical findings. Duke's Ed Hammond argued that an NPI would have a much lower error rate than the 2-18% error rates encountered using current matching algorithms. The Covid-19 pandemic highlights the need for an NPI since public health entities need longitudinal data to inform national response. Others stressed that while an NPI would link patients with a unique number to identify them, that's not necessarily enough to authenticate a patient.

Patient matching is a complex issue but removing the federal funding ban on unique patient identifiers would be an important step towards achieving interoperability and improving patient care.

TMR's Take - America has made some progress towards more integrated patient information over the past decade but lags far behind other major democracies. In France, interoperability is ensured via a chip on patients' health cards. Hospital-based and office-based professionals and patients have a unique electronic identifier. In Germany, electronic medical chip cards have been used nationwide since 2015.

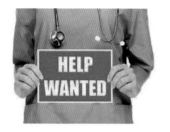

New AAMC Report Confirms Growing Physician Shortage, 6/26/2020

TMR Topline™ - In its sixth annual study, The Complexities of Physician Supply and Demand: Projections from 2018-2033, the American Association of Medical Colleges projects an estimated shortage of between 54,100 and 139,000 physicians by 2033. The study was conducted in 2019 prior to the pandemic.

TMR's Take - The AAMC's latest projection of physician shortages by 2025 is more than 40% higher than its 2017 estimate. More than 30% of America's physicians are over 55. To attract more Americans to practice medicine, the high cost of a medical education must be addressed, and incentives need to be provided to correct the primary care/specialists imbalance. Other issues to be addressed include stress of dealing with private insurance pre-authorization requirements and the burdensome aspects of electronic health records on physician practices

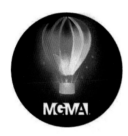

Pandemic may pound lopsided physician pay model into shape, by Ginger Christ, Modern Healthcare, 7/18/20

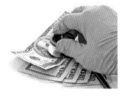

Covid-19 will have lasting effects on providers, including how they operate and how they're paid, by Dr. Halee Fischer-Wright, Modern Healthcare, 8/3/20

TMR Topline™ - The article and subsequent op-ed provide an interesting point-counterpoint on the pandemic's impact on how physicians are paid. The article describes the dramatic effect that the pandemic has had on physician pay. Medical specialties that are normally in high demand were furloughed or saw pay cuts and layoffs as elective procedures were reduced or restricted. Compounding the effect, patients deferred seeking care to avoid exposure to the virus. As a result, procedure-driven specialist income fell dramatically. Experts estimate that 18% of physicians who have treated Covid-19 patients have been furloughed or experienced pay cuts while 30% of those not treating these patients had their pay reduced or were furloughed by their health systems.

Prior to the pandemic, physician compensation grew by 2% to 3% annually with specialists earning substantially more than generalists. From 2016 to 2019 surgical specialties increased by more than 8% and family practice and internal medicine increased from 2% to 7%.

Dr. Fischer-Wright, President and CEO of the Medical Group Management Association, points out that healthcare has been one of the hardest hit segments of the economy. The pandemic's impacts on patient care were unanticipated and could be a factor for many years. In addition to patients delaying preventative and non-emergency care, the rapid adoption of telehealth changed the way providers will be paid in the future. Dr. Fischer-Wright believes more healthcare providers will be needed as the U.S. population ages. The treatment challenges experienced during the pandemic further compound the stress on healthcare workers, suffering burnout at alarming rates. MGMA's report on the financial impact of the virus found that, on average, practices have experienced a 55% decrease in revenue and a 60% decrease in patient volume.

2019 was a decent year for most doctors according to Modern Healthcare's 27th annual Physician Compensation Survey. The 2019 salary increases were largely due to productivity gains. However, 1.4 million healthcare workers were furloughed in April and larger health systems are beginning to realign their volume-based compensation models. Both authors believe that many health systems will begin to explore value-based compensation while others will work to rebuild their patient volumes while working to reduce their costs.

TMR's Take - The pandemic has highlighted many long-standing problems of the U.S. healthcare system, including the imbalance between primary and specialty care, financing mechanisms broken beyond easy repair and a focus on curing, not preventing, disease. America needs to place more emphasis on public health and preventive care and address the growing shortage of primary care physicians. The U.S. is the sole OECD member that fails to recognize universal access to healthcare as a basic human right, not a privilege for those that can afford it. The Eichhorn-Hutchinson Allcare plan provides a framework for a universal healthcare system that provides choice along with a public option and reduces administrative waste, drug costs and medically related bankruptcies.

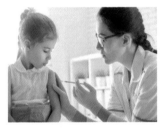

Pharmacists in 50 states can give childhood shots to prevent future outbreaks, officials say, by Mike Stobbe, Associated Press, 8/20/20

TMR Topline™ - Exercising his emergency powers, HHS Secretary Alex Azar has temporarily preempted restrictions in 22 states starting this fall. Pharmacists in all 50 states will be allowed to vaccinate children over 3 years old without a doctor's prescription. According to a CDC report, orders for childhood vaccines from doctors' offices plummeted in late March and April. Most childhood vaccinations are given in a doctor's office. The CDC reported that only 7% were administered in pharmacies in 2018. Azar stated, *"It is critical that children have easy access to the pediatric vaccinations to enable them to get back to school as schools reopen."*

TMR's Take - Americans tend to trust their pharmacists, so Azar's directive preempting restrictions in 22 states is a welcome move.

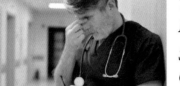

The Biggest Challenges Facing Physicians, by Todd Shryock, Medical Economics 8/7/20

Survey: Physician Burnout on the Rise, by Maria Calstellucci, Modern Healthcare 9/21/20

TMR Topline™ Recently the American Osteopathic Association (AOA) did a national survey of small and mid-size practices to learn how the pandemic has affected them. In an interview with Medical Economics, AOA President Dr. Thomas Ely, DO discussed survey results, the pandemic, burnout, and financial challenges doctors are facing. The pandemic has created two vastly different realities for physicians. They either are swamped with Covid-19 patients or struggling financially because patients are afraid to come in for their appointments or elective procedures have been postponed.

Of the practices responding, 95% experienced a decline in revenue, 40% estimate that 2020 physician revenue will half what it was in 2019, and three quarters believe that they will need financial support to be able to continue to provide quality patient care. There are widespread reports that health care providers are showing significant rates of post-traumatic stress, anxiety, insomnia, and depression. Dr. Ely urges that anyone on the front lines in need of support should reach out to the physician support line at www.physiciansupportline.com. It's a free and confidential service to support the mental health of doctors and medical students,

A Physicians Foundation August survey of 2,300 physicians found that because of the pandemic, those surveyed who reported burnout increased from 40% to 58% since the 2018 survey. Since the pandemic began *"taking care of patients has become much more difficult,"* said Dr. Gary Price, President of the Physicians Foundation. Physicians in coronavirus hot spots report exhaustion or feelings of inadequacy.

Some private practices have been forced to close or furlough staff due to lost revenue. The survey also found 38% of physicians want to retire in the next year, including 21% of those 45 or younger. In the 2018 survey 17% said they plan to retire in the next one to three years. Dr. Price found this alarming given that the average age of the physician workforce is over 50 with a shortage is predicted in the years ahead. *"If the pandemic accelerated what already is a looming problem, it would be disastrous as far as patients' access to care."*

TMR's Take - The pandemic has put added stress on physicians while dramatically reducing practice income for many. With a significant physician shortage looming, the U.S. needs to find imaginative ways to reduce physician burnout and provide financial support.

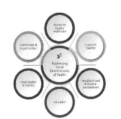

RWJBarnabas Health launches tech-enabled social determinants of health program, by Mallory Hackett, Healthcare Finance News, 10/14/20

TMR Topline™ - RWJBarnabas Health is collaborating with NowPow and ConsejoSano to refer and connect patients to community-based services in addressing the social determinants of health (SDOH). The goal is to assess patients' risk factors for chronic disease by removing the stigma around questioning housing, safety, and nutrition. After the initial screening, the Health Beyond the Hospital program uses NowPow's community referral platform to connect people with services personalized to meet their health and social needs based on age, gender, eligibility, location, primary language, and insurance coverage. ConsejoSano's patient engagement platform uses culturally and linguistically tailored tools to serve patients using the communication method that works best for everyone, engaging patients through text, phone call, email, or mail in over 22 languages.

America has worse health outcomes than other OECD members including higher infant mortality rates and lower life expectancy. The Covid-19 pandemic is affecting marginalized groups at higher rates. A 2016 Health Affairs article found that effectively alleviating health disparities requires programs that focus on early childhood education, urban planning and community development, housing, income enhancements and employment. Independence Blue Cross and Signify Health launched a similar initiative recently called Community Link, designed to break the barriers between social and clinical care by helping people gain access to nonmedical health services such as food, housing, transportation.

After completing the pilot program, Health Beyond the Hospital will be expanded across the system. According to RWJ Barnabas Health CEO Barry Ostrowsky, *"80% of all health outcomes are due to social, behavioral, and environmental factors that are the social determinants of health… The timely interventions made possible by Health Beyond the Hospital will create a spiral that will positively impact the well-being of our patients and all of those caring for patients across our community."*

TMR's Take –The World Health Organization defines health as *"a state of complete physical, mental and **social** well-being."* Health systems that succeed in providing better care while improving healthy behaviors in the communities they serve will lower the per capita costs of care and produce better outcomes on the key health indicators. Full disclosure: The Editor is an Honorary Trustee at an RWJBarnabas Health affiliated hospital.

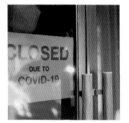

Thousands of Doctors' Offices Buckle Under Financial Stress of COVID, by Laura Ungar, Kaiser Health News, 11/30/20

TMR Topline™ - A wave of Covid-related closures is reducing access to care in areas already short on primary care doctors. Recent research by the Physicians Foundation suggests that 8% (roughly 16,0000 physician practices) have closed due to the stress of the pandemic. A late September survey from the Primary Care Collaborative and the Green Center found that 7% of primary care practices were unsure they could stay open past December without financial assistance. Prior to the pandemic, America faced a shortage of 15,000 primary care physicians; federal data shows that 82 million Americans live in primary care *"health professional shortage areas."* Experts are concerned that patients managing chronic conditions are the biggest losers when such closures occur.

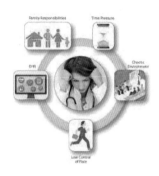

Healthcare workers experiencing burnout, stress due to COVID-19 pandemic, by Jeff Lagasse, Associate Editor, Healthcare Finance, 12/8/20

TMR Topline™ - Two recent surveys confirm that the pandemic is taking an enormous toll on the mental health of healthcare workers and contributing to anxiety, stress, depression, loneliness, and other concerns. A survey of more than 1,000 healthcare workers conducted by Mental Health America (MHA) from June to September found 93% experiencing stress, 86% experiencing anxiety, 77% reporting frustration, 76% reporting exhaustion and burnout, and 75% stating they were overwhelmed. They also worried about exposing their families to Covid-19: nearly half were worried about exposing their spouse, partner, or older family member, and 75% about exposing their child.

Over 82% reported experiencing emotional exhaustion followed by trouble with sleep (70%), physical exhaustion (68%) and work-related dread (63%). In a survey by a Berkshire Hathaway Specialty Insurance division, 84% reported feeling at least mildly burned out from work, with 18% feeling totally burned out. The top five stresses that respondents shared were fear of getting Covid-19; long hours/shifts; the general state of the world; fear of spreading the coronavirus; and family issues and responsibilities. Nearly half have considered either retiring, quitting their jobs, or changing their careers altogether, while the same number say that their mental health has deteriorated. In summary, both surveys found healthcare workers stressed out and stretched too thin.

TMR's Take - It's time to reinvent how American healthcare is delivered: with 25% of the population already living in areas with primary care shortages and practices closing, and most of the healthcare workforce experiencing burnout, lots needs to change. Telehealth and workplace redesign are part of the solution as is providing mental health support, but more is needed.

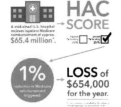

Medicare Cuts Payment to 774 Hospitals Over Patient Complications, by Jordan Rau, Kaiser Health News, 2/19/21

TMR Topline™ - The Hospital-Acquired Condition Reduction Program is penalizing 774 hospitals for having the highest rates of patient infections or other potentially avoidable medical complications between mid-2017 and 2019 (pre-pandemic). They will lose 1% of their Medicare payments over 12 months beginning 10/1/21 for being in the top quarter for preventable conditions like sepsis, central line infections, catheter associated UTIs, etc. Created by the ACA to motivate hospitals to protect patients from harm, the program is in its 7th year. According to the CDC, on any given day, 1 in 31 patients has an infection that was contracted during the stay. The American Hospital Association describes the penalties as *"a game of chance"* based on *"badly flawed"* measures. Renowned hospitals penalized this year include LA's Cedars-Sinai, New York-Presbyterian, and Vanderbilt.

TMR's Take –The AHA has a valid point – the data should be risk adjusted. Here in New Jersey, all three Level 1 Trauma Centers are penalized virtually every year. That said, both articles reinforce the need for comprehensive healthcare reform with robust public health and disease prevention programs. America's hospitals excel at treating illness, but face infection prevention challenges daily.

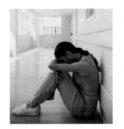

American Nursing is having a Crisis, by Theresa Brown, New York Times, 2/28/21

TMR Topline™ - Author of *"The Shift: One Nurse, Twelve Hours, Four Patients' Lives."*, Theresa Brown's heart-rending interviews with six veteran nurses throughout the U.S. are intermingled with evidence of the growing shortage of these vital caregivers. The Bureau of Labor Statistics projects that 176,000 new nurses will be needed annually yet nursing schools don't have enough faculty to expand the nursing work force. Add to that the numbers of nurses who are beyond burnout due to the pandemic.

Brown cites research that Covid nurses are now suffering from *"moral injury,"* a term typically applied to combat soldiers. She quotes an El Paso ICU nurse: *"It's moral injury when I leave a hospital bursting at the seams and all the bars and stores are full of people."* Another ICU veteran is studying to become a nurse practitioner. *"I'm going into primary care to keep people out of the hospital,"* she said. 'We never had enough nurses.*"*

A 2020 report from HFMA shows that having enough nurses in hospitals can save money, yet 36 of America's 60 largest hospital chains have laid off, furloughed, or cut the pay of staff members to save money during the pandemic.

Brown calls for changes in the profession that include finding creative ways to bring more nurses into the work force, adding faculty for nursing schools and making them more affordable.

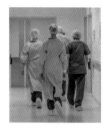

Average nursing home nursing staff turnover exceeds 100%, report finds, by Ginger Christ, Modern Healthcare, 3/1/21

TMR Topline™ - Health Affairs has released a recent study reporting that the average rate of nursing home staff turnover is more than 100% per year. The turnover rate for registered nurses was 140.7% while the rate for licensed practical nurses and certified nursing assistants was 114.1%. Ashvin Gandhi, assistant professor at UCLA Anderson School of Management, coauthor of the report, said *"We see fairly clear evidence that higher turnover rates tend to be associated with a lot of factors that are associated with worse quality of care."*

Nursing homes with higher levels of Medicaid residents had higher turnover. These facilities may also pay less because Medicaid reimbursement is lower than Medicare or private insurance payment. As a result of the high turnover rate in nursing homes, the authors recommend nursing staff turnover rates should be included on the CMS Nursing Home Compare Quality Rating System. With turnover data now available, researchers will be able to look at how those rates relate to health outcomes. Prospective patients and employees will have more complete data available to evaluate facilities.

TMR's Take –These two articles are a clarion call for action to avert an impending critical shortage of caregivers for the rapidly aging "Baby Boomer" population. The alternative is unacceptable.

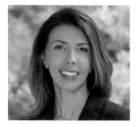

Healthcare leaders can't go wrong if we keep the patient at the center of every decision, by Carrie Owen Plietz, Modern Healthcare, 3/22/21

TMR Topline™ - The author is incoming Chair of the American College of Healthcare Executives and President of Kaiser Permanente Northern California. Her commentary is a reflection on integrity, *"the fundamental value that is one of our profession's most essential attributes."* Noting that *"it has been critical in our ability to navigate the Covid-19 pandemic,"* she calls for *"reaffirming our own commitment to professional integrity."*

Ms. Plietz equates the meaning of integrity with advice she received from her mentor: *""If you make every decision with the patient at the center of that decision, you'll never make a bad decision."* Her advice is to *"work intentionally every day on maintaining ethical standards in every decision, communication, huddle and personal interaction. In the same way high-reliability organizations hold safety huddles, start meetings with a mission moment and talk about good catches."* While it's not easy to take the high road in all cases, she recommends *"Remaining centered on what is best for the patient and letting it guide our decisions and our relationships with our teams and communities, is our North Star."*

TMR's Take –Ms. Plietz's sound advice resonates with the Editor, who serves on a hospital Board where every meeting begins with a Safety Story and decisions are reached through the prism of what's best for the patients we serve.

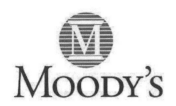

NFP hospital profitability plummeted in 2020 despite expense mitigation strategies, Moody's reports, by Nick Hut, HFMA, 3/31/21

TMR Topline™ - The suspension of elective procedures and slow pace of patient volume recovery were key factors in the declining profitability of not-for-profit (NFP) hospitals in 2020 according to Moody's Investor Services, the credit rating agency. The median operating margin for hospitals and health systems was 0.5%, down from 2.4% in FY19. Management *"curtailed labor expenses and saw some reduction in supply costs as volumes declined, particularly in elective surgeries,"* Moody's reported, even though costs of personal protective equipment increased significantly. Moody's outlook for the NFP healthcare sector this year is negative.

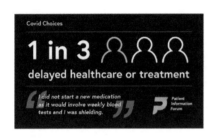

From Rotten Teeth to Advanced Cancer, Patients Feel the Effects of Treatment Delays, by Bruce Alpert, Kaiser Health News, 4/20/21

TMR Topline™ - As vaccinated Americans resume routine medical care, doctors and dentists are seeing the realities of pandemic-delayed preventive and emergency care. Along with stress related ailments they are finding more advanced cancer and cardiac disease and rotting and damaged teeth. Dr. Brian Rah, cardiology department chair at Montana's Billings Clinic, was concerned; some patients arrived hours after feeling chest pains because they were afraid of contracting Covid-19 by going to the hospital. *"For a heart attack patient, the first hour is known as the golden hour,"* Rah said. After that, the likelihood of death and/or a lifelong reduction in activities and health increases.

Detroit pediatrician Dr. Gerald Mosby finds his young patients are suffering more stress, depression, and weight gain than before the pandemic. Dr. J.P. Valin, chief clinical officer at SCL Health of Colorado and Montana, said he is *"kept awake at night"* by delays in important medical tests. *"People put off routine breast examinations, and there are going to be some cancers hiding that are not going to be identified, potentially delaying intervention."* He expressed concern that patients with appendicitis symptoms like abdominal pain, fever and nausea aren't seeking timely treatment. A burst appendix involves more risk and a longer hospital stay. Arkansas optometrist Matthew Jones is seeing much more eyestrain *"because people are spending so much time in front of a computer screen."*

A recent American Dental Association survey found that more than 70% of member dentists reported an increase in patients grinding or clenching their teeth since Covid. More than 60% reported an increase in other stress-related conditions, such as chipped and cracked teeth. Some providers report nearing pre-Covid office visit levels; others still face Covid resistance. Neville Gupta of Gupta Gastro in Brooklyn and Far Rockaway, New York said. *"Our patients are still avoiding getting the care they need, no matter the safety precautions in place."*

TMR's Take - Until America achieves herd immunity, many will continue to defer care, likely resulting in higher mortality rates and billions in costs.

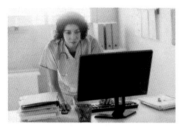

Telehealth can increase nurses' workloads, study finds, by Alex Kacik, Modern Healthcare, 4/30/21

TMR Topline™ - A new study reports that while telehealth can increase access to care, it also has the potential to increase nursing workloads. A University of Missouri study reports that nurses performed about twice as many activities with telehealth patients when compared to in-person patients. Their analysis of nearly 800 nursing activities performed for Type 2 diabetes and hypertension patients found that in-person visits had follow-ups every three months, while telehealth patients submitted glucose and blood pressure levels many times a week.

The study's lead author Chelsea Howland said, *"For participants who had an in-home monitoring system, there were more nursing activities related to diabetes and health education, more medication adjustments and more follow-ups with nurses."* Care for U.S. diabetes and hypertension patients costs about $380 billion a year. Telehealth advocates hope that it can ease the burden of chronic diseases. Telehealth has demonstrated its convenience and flexibility for patients during the COVID-19 pandemic, but there are concerns that it could lead to redundant care, make health disparities worse and lead to more fraud.

Concerned that additional telehealth workload for nurses could cause an already stretched and short-staffed nursing population to leave the field, Howland said. *"There should be some additional training in how to integrate the technology into the workflow."*

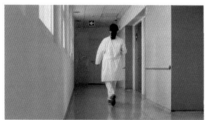

Women in healthcare are at a breaking point—and they're leaving, by Shefali Luthra and Chabeli Carrazana, The 19th, 5/17/21

TMR Topline™ - Women in healthcare today face enormous pandemic-related challenges, including memories of the thousands of healthcare workers and patients that have perished. Many say the coronavirus crisis caused them to leave the workforce or dramatically scale back their professional commitment. Many do not know if they will ever return. At least 1/3 have experienced burnout. In April 2020, women lost or left more than 1.5 million healthcare jobs, 12% of all women employed in healthcare. With the recovery underway, women have been much slower to return to employment than men. In March, there were 480,000 open positions usually filled by women compared with 28,000 for men.

The Covid caregiving challenges fell largely on women healthcare workers who earn the least. Certified nursing assistant Kenya Blackburn would have been responsible for about five patients a shift 20 years ago. At the pandemic's peak, she was assigned as many as 30 patients in an eight-hour shift, earning $15.00/hour. Many of the pandemic healthcare job losses were concentrated in lower-paying settings like home care and long-term care.

CNAs like Blackburn are 82% female earning an average of $14.82/hour. Home health aides average $13.02/hour and are 90% female.

Currently, just over 50% of medical school students are women. After completing residencies, women are more likely to leave medicine due to burnout, harassment and pay inequities, and nearly 40% leave their jobs or take part-time positions within six years. Women leaving healthcare could pose serious challenges for the nation as the population ages and more Americans need skilled nursing or home care. *"These care and healthcare occupations are absolutely critical to supporting our entire country, and to supporting the people who are most vulnerable — who are sick, who are children and who are elderly, who need this serious and intensive medical care,"* said Diana Boesch, a women's economic policy analyst at the Center for American Progress, *"If we don't support the workers in those jobs, we will continue to face a crisis of care and a crisis of healthcare."* President Biden has proposed plans that could alleviate some of these challenges. He has called for improved access to childcare and for reforms that would pay home care workers a $15 minimum wage, and would provide opportunities for advancement.

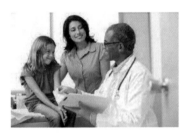

A Primary Care Physician for Every American, Science Panel Urges, by Noam K. Levy, Kaiser Health News, 5/4/21

TMR Topline™ - In an urgently worded report, the National Academies of Sciences, Engineering and Medicine recommend that all Americans select a primary care provider or be assigned one, and that Medicare and Medicaid shift money to primary care and away from the medical specialties that have long commanded the biggest fees in the U.S. system.

It comes as internists, family doctors and pediatricians nationwide struggle with the economic fallout of the coronavirus pandemic and calls for a broad recognition that primary care is a *"common good"* akin to public education. According to OECD data, about 5% of U.S. healthcare spending goes to primary care, compared with 14% in other wealthy nations.

Research shows that robust primary care systems save money, improve people's health, and even save lives. Europeans with chronic illnesses reported significantly better health if they lived in a country with a robust primary care system. The report urges new initiatives to build more health centers, especially in underserved areas, and to expand primary care teams, including nurse practitioners, pharmacists, and mental health specialists. Medicare, Medicaid, and employers that provide their workers with health benefits should ask their members to declare a primary care provider.

One top performing system, Kaiser-Permanente, has long made primary care central. Co-chair of the Committee that produced the report Dr. Robert Phillips said: *"If we increase the supply of primary care, more people and more communities will be healthier, and no other part of health care can make this claim."*

TMR's Take: An independent review ordered by the World Health Organization found that Covid-19 was *"a preventable disaster,"* exposing dangerous failings on both the national and international scale. The *"preventable disaster"* leaves American healthcare facing a perfect storm as it recovers: a critical need to expand primary care when women are leaving healthcare and telehealth may increase nurses' workloads. Dr. Yalda Jabbarpour, a primary care doctor who studies family medicine policy said *"It's really important that our healthcare system revamps and thinks about what women in the workforce need. The pandemic has brought that to light."* **TMR** agrees.

The Fastest-Growing U.S. States Have the Worst Health Care, by David Blumenthal and David C. Radley, Harvard Business Review, 6/2/21

TMR Topline™ - The op-ed by David Blumenthal and David Radley of the Commonwealth Fund summarized the Fund's annual state rankings, finding that the U.S. states with the fastest-growing population score worst when it comes to the quality of their residents' health and access to care. The fastest-growing states in terms of population over the last decade, including Texas (42), Florida (41), and Georgia (46), consistently rank last when it comes to health and health care. Low-ranking states have large numbers of uninsured adults, high levels of premature death from treatable conditions, less investment in public health, too many people with mental illness unable to get the care they need, and residents facing mounting insurance costs. Texas has the highest uninsured rate in the U.S. and the largest number of residents who said they skipped health care they needed due to cost. Georgia has one of the highest rates of premature death from treatable conditions and one of the highest rates of infant mortality. The authors argue that the subsidies included in the American Rescue Plan should be made permanent, stating that health insurance coverage is the most important determinant of access to health care.

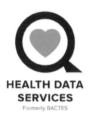

Healthiest states in the U.S. during the 2020 pandemic were in the Northeast, by Kerry Breen, NBC News, 5/25/21

TMR Topline™ - Digital health company Sharecare's Community Well-Being Index looks at social determinants of health like access to health care, food, housing, transportation and personal health risk factors including physical health, community and social bonds, financial management skills and strength of purpose in daily life. For the first time in several years, Hawaii didn't top the list, finishing second after Massachusetts, followed by New Jersey, Maryland and New York. Residents in the top-ranked states have lower-than-average individual health risk factors and say that they enjoy supportive relationships with other people, have the tools to manage and increase their financial security regardless of income, and have access to high-quality health care and jobs. For the second year in a row, Mississippi finished last, ahead of Arkansas, New Mexico, West Virginia and Kentucky. Researchers from Sharecare and Boston University's School of Public Health assessed 450,000 respondents from 50 states.

TMR's Take - The ranking criteria differ but Mississippi was last in both. **TMR** is proud that Sharecare ranks its home state of New Jersey third in the U.S. Sandwiched between New York and Philadelphia, the Garden State's robust healthcare system and social services safety net often is overlooked. In an intriguing anomaly, 9 of Sharecare's top 10 states voted for Biden; 9 of the bottom 10 voted for Trump in the 2020 Presidential election.

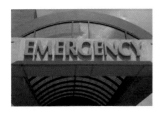

ED visits decline during pandemic as patients access other avenues for care, by Mari Devereaux, Modern Healthcare, 6/8/21

TMR Topline™ - Emergency Department visits have dropped significantly since the start of the Covid-19 pandemic for a host of reasons. Among them:

- people interacting less and going out less, leading to lower numbers of accidents, illnesses and infectious diseases;
- the increased number of deaths among nursing home patients and those with chronic medical problems due to Covid-19;
- many new options for patients to see a physician or seek care using their computers, phones and access points for telehealth; and
- alternatives to ED visits enabled by payment structures that allowed telehealth to expand rapidly during the pandemic.

Kaufman Hall noted while there has been some recovery in ED visits since the early months of the pandemic, levels are still about 15-20% lower than prior averages.

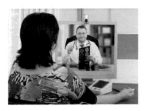

Persistent myths could send telehealth back to pre-pandemic regulation, by Krista Drobac, Modern Healthcare, 7/2/21

TMR Topline™ - Executive Director of the Alliance for Connected Care Krista Drobac is concerned that some persistent myths could derail the prospects for long-term telehealth coverage:

1. **Lifting Medicare telehealth restrictions will cost the program money.** Concerns about excess utilization have not materialized. Telehealth filled in for office visits during peak social distancing periods and declined as people went back to the doctor's office. Conversely, telehealth consultations from March to July of 2020 successfully diverted millions of dollars of Skilled Nursing Facility transfers.

2. **Patients aren't seeing their own doctors.** A large study of patients' telehealth behavior during the pandemic found 83% of seniors saw their own provider or a colleague; only 1% saw a virtual provider that they didn't know.

3. **Telehealth is uniquely subject to fraud.** Press releases from the DoJ have created a false impression that telehealth is highly vulnerable to criminal fraud. However, most dealt with various telemarketing scams, not telehealth.

4. **In-person relationship requirements are necessary to mitigate excessive cost and fraud.** Requiring patients to first complete an in-person visit creates a barrier to care for the homebound and those in underserved areas. All 50 state legislatures have abolished in-person requirements for telehealth visits, and the AMA has said a physician-patient relationship can be established by telehealth.

5. **The Biden administration has the authority to make the telehealth changes permanent**. Congress granted the authority that federal agencies needed to allow Medicare to cover telehealth and that will expire with the end of the public health emergency.

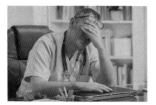

Addressing the 'public health crisis' of healthcare worker burnout, by Ginger Christ, Modern Healthcare, 6/22/21

TMR Topline™ - The pandemic didn't create staff burnout in healthcare workers; it exacerbated it. A survey by Mental Health America during the pandemic found 93% of healthcare workers surveyed said they had experienced stress in the past three months, 86% reported anxiety, 77% reported frustration, 76% reported exhaustion and burnout, and 75% said they were overwhelmed. Industry experts suggest giving clinicians more flexibility in their schedules and reducing their administrative burden. They recommend parity in payment for mental health services and say health systems need to intensify efforts to eliminate the stigma around mental health issues. Some see telehealth as a way to improve doctors' work-life balance, if done correctly. Others look to technology to reduce the burden on clinicians by automating tedious tasks like data entry. North Carolina's Novant Health launched a *"Thriving Together"* platform last year to address the issue that combines the internal resources available to employees to thrive in their personal lives and at work.

TMR's Take - Burnout is a critical issue that must be addressed, particularly removing the stigma around mental health issues. The article describes a broad range of approaches being taken by health systems across the U.S. to deal with the issue.

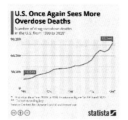

'It's Huge, It's Historic, It's Unheard-of': Drug Overdose Deaths Spike, by Josh Katz and Margot Sanger-Katz, New York Times, 7/14/21

TMR Topline™ - As the Covid pandemic raged, drug abuse deaths rose 30% to more than 93,000 in 2020, disproportionately among the young. Deaths rose in every state but New Hampshire and South Dakota, with the greatest increases in the South and West. A Times analysis estimates that the drug deaths represent 3.5 million years of life compared to 5.5 million for the 375,000 Covid deaths. The pandemic's disruption to outreach and treatment facilities and increased social isolation contributed to the increase as did fentanyls becoming entrenched in the nation's drug supply. Fentanyls are easier to manufacture and ship than traditional heroin with higher potency. The pandemic brought some policy changes that may have saved lives such as allowing people enrolled in methadone treatment to take doses home with them, instead of having to visit a clinic each day. Regulators also made it easier for people to seek medical care through telemedicine.

TMR's Take - TMR supports efforts to change treatment policies to allow people enrolled in methadone treatment to take doses home with them instead of having to be at a clinic each day and the expanded use of telemedicine for these patients.

CHAPTER 6

Insurance: Too Many Plans, Too Much Overhead, Too Complicated

A MERICA'S UNIQUE BLEND OF PUBLIC AND PRIVATE SOURCES OF HEALTH INSURANCE COVERAGE HAS BEEN A major contributor to the highest per capita health care costs in the world – as well as a major cause of provider frustration and burnout. It's REALLY complicated!

Overall, nearly half of Americans receive their health insurance coverage through a government program such as Medicare, Medicaid and the Children's Health Insurance Program (CHIP), the Veterans Administration, or the Indian Health Service. According to the Centers for Medicare and Medicaid Services (CMS), more than 80 million people were enrolled and receiving full benefits from the Medicaid and CHIP programs by the end of January 2021.

With more than 63 million beneficiaries, Medicare continues to expand as 10,000 baby boomers a day become eligible when they turn 65. In addition to those over 65, Medicare also covers certain American adults with disabilities and those with end stage renal disease (ESRD). While the federal government sets Medicare policies, the program is administered by private contractors who compete vigorously for the business. Thus, despite the program's complexity, its administrative costs average 2% of expenditures according to the Kaiser Family Foundation.

Medicaid is a federal/state partnership administered by state governments following broad national guidelines established by federal statutes, regulations, and policies. Primary beneficiaries include pregnant women, children and low-income adults. Like Medicare, Medicaid programs are administered by private contractors who compete vigorously for the business.

Private health insurance is the predominant source of health insurance coverage in the United States. According to the Congressional Research Service, in 2019 these markets covered an estimated 179 million individuals (55.4% of the U.S. population) and 42 million individuals (13.1% of the U.S. population), respectively.

While this represents the largest number of insured, the extent and amount of coverage provided varies widely, and an estimated 40 million Americans are underinsured.

The number of Americans, who lack health insurance coverage varies, but was estimated to be 30 million midway through 2020, up from 28 million in 2016. In 2010, prior to the passage of the Affordable Care Act (ACA), 48 million Americans were uninsured.

Surveys have found that most Americans who have private health insurance coverage are satisfied with their plans and would like to keep them even if there was a universal healthcare plan like Medicare for All that as proposed by Senator Bernie Sanders. Their experience tells them that they are aligned with their health insurance provider because they are confident that coverage will be there when they need it.

On the other hand, health insurers design benefit plans that are aligned with the needs of their customers. For group coverage, that's the employer, not the individual or families receiving the coverage. Over the past 20 years, that has resulted in the growth of high-deductible health plans (HDHPs) that have shifted a significant part of the expense from the employer to the insured employee and family.

The private insurance industry (especially the for-profit companies) is an excellent example of perverse incentives in action. There's an adage among providers: "*Insurers love to collect premiums but hate to pay claims.*" Profits are higher when fewer claims are paid. As a result, America's private health insurers have become extremely adept at finding creative ways to delay services (e.g., prior authorization required) and to defer or deny provider claims. In addition to increasing administrative expenses, these tactics are a significant contributing factor in provider burnout.

Prior to the passage of the ACA, there were no limits on what insurers could spend on sales, general and administrative expenses. The ACA requires that large insurers spend 85% of premiums on medical care and small insurers 80% (the medical loss ratio). Compare that to Medicare's 98% of premium on medical care and it's evident that major savings could be achieved if insurers were required to compete with the Medicare program. Higher medical loss ratios translate into lower healthcare costs. For other OECD member countries with universal healthcare systems, it's 95% or higher.

Like the pharmaceutical industry, insurers have one of the most powerful lobbying organizations in Washington, America's Health Insurance Plans (AHIP).

The 23 articles summarized in this chapter cover topics including:

- The challenges of insurance coverage for the pandemic induced recession
- Prior Authorization issues for payers and providers
- Federal efforts to improve access to health insurance
- Efforts to address the many challenges of private health insurance

Insurance coverage in the United States was complicated before the Covid-19 pandemic began. The pandemic highlighted many longstanding issues that should be addressed to provide better access to care at lower prices for all Americans.

Insurance Coverage Three Minute Reads

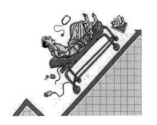

COVID – 19 Could Mean $251B Spike in Health Costs, California Says, by Adam Lidgett for Law360.com, 3/23/20

TMR Topline™ - In the first study of its kind, Covered California, the state's healthcare marketplace, projects that the Covid-19 pandemic could increase healthcare costs in the national commercial insurance market by as much as $251 billion over the next 12 months. Many of the 170 million Americans who secure coverage in the private insurance market may not get the care they need. Absent Federal intervention individuals and businesses will likely see increased premiums and reduced benefits. They recommend Federal intervention to provide monetary support for people below the poverty line and a program to limit costs for self-insured companies and insurers. Covered California has opened a special pandemic enrollment period through the end of June for California's uninsured population.

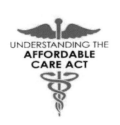

Eligibility for ACA Health Coverage Following Job Loss, by Rachel Garfield, Gary Claxton, Anthony Damico, and Larry Levitt, Kaiser Family Foundation, 5/13/20

TMR Topline™ - Between March 1st and May 2nd, more than 31 million people had filed for unemployment insurance. Job loss carries the risk of loss of health insurance for people who were receiving health coverage as a benefit through their employer. This study estimates their eligibility for ACA coverage, including Medicaid and marketplace subsidies, as well as private coverage as a dependent. Most people who lose ESI due to job loss will be eligible for ACA assistance either through Medicaid or subsidized marketplace coverage. However, some people will fall outside the reach of the ACA, particularly in January 2021 when UI benefits cease for many, and some adults fall into the Medicaid coverage gap due to state decisions not to expand coverage under the ACA.

TMR's Take - The KFF is a trusted source for credible information and the May survey results are disturbing. **TMR** will continue to monitor.

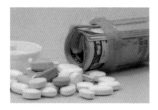

Major Insurers Pledge $55 Million to Try to Lower Generic Drug Prices, by Katie Thomas for the New York Times, 1/23/20

TMR Topline™ - The Blue Cross Blue Shield Association and 18 of its members have agreed to invest $55 million to develop less expensive versions of high-priced generic drugs that have limited competition. The participating organizations insure over 40 million Americans. Drug prices have continued to climb and are the fastest growing cost segment of U.S. health care at $429 billion. Absent of competitive pressure or federal regulation, drug costs are likely to continue to climb. The Blues will partner with Civica Rx, a nonprofit that currently sells generic drugs to hospitals and health systems, and plan to start with 7 to 10 drugs that they hope to bring to market in 2022.

TMR's Take - Civica was created in 2018 by a group of charitable foundations and hospital systems to address the many shortages of essential drugs that hospitals were experiencing. Civica's first sales of 18 drugs occurred last fall.

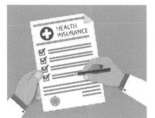

How the COVID-19 Recession Could Affect Health Insurance Coverage, by Bowen Garrett, Anuj Gangopadhyaya, Urban Institute, 5/4/20

TMR Topline™ - Thirty million workers filed initial unemployment claims between March 15 and April 25. The report presents national and state-level estimates of coverage changes if unemployment rates rise from pre-crisis levels (around 3.5 percent nationally) to 15 percent, 20 percent, or 25 percent. For each unemployment level, it provides a base case scenario of coverage changes and a high scenario, derived from two different estimation methods. In the base scenario an estimated 25 million people will lose employer sponsored insurance (ESI) coverage at 20% unemployment. Of them, 12 million would gain Medicaid coverage, 6 million would gain marketplace or other private coverage, and 7 million would become uninsured. In the high scenario, an estimated 43 million people would lose ESI coverage.

TMR's Take - Prior to the pandemic, 160 million Americans received health insurance coverage through their employer. As both previous articles indicate, an unprecedented number of Americans will lose ESI coverage during the pandemic. There will be significant lapses in coverage, and many will become uninsured.

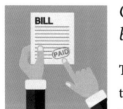

Congress said COVID-19 tests should be free—but who's paying?, by Blake Farmer, Kaiser Health News, 5/22/20

TMR Topline™ - When Congress enacted the Families First Coronavirus Response Act and the CARES Act, its stated intent was that Covid-19 testing would be covered and there would be no copays and no out-of-pocket costs for patients. However, it is unclear whether the laws apply to self-funded plans that may be exempt under ERISA. Many companies with such plans are operating as if they are exempt from the rules.

Compounding the confusion, the Congressional mandate does not apply to related services that the patient may have received during testing. As a result, many Covid-19 testing centers are holding off on billing, concerned about consumer outrage when a surprise bill hits their mailbox. Many are holding back billing for Covid-19 testing services due to the confusion, depriving providers of needed cash flow during the crisis.

TMR's Take - between millions losing ESI coverage and the confusion over Covid-19 testing coverage, providers are facing a billing and collection nightmare that likely will take years to unravel.

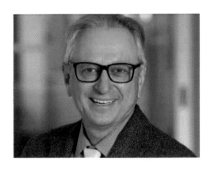

The payer-provider disconnect, by Merrill Goozner, Modern Healthcare, 5/18/20

TMR Topline™ - Goozner is a keen observer of American healthcare and its flaws and failings. In this perceptive editorial, he dissects the paradox of insurers doing just fine while thousands of healthcare providers face financial ruin and tens of millions of Americans are losing insurance coverage. As for America's for-profit insurers, first-quarter results were just fine, and full year earnings estimates were left unchanged.

The first three bailout bills included $175 million for providers but included no rules on the money's use and there is widespread concern that small physician practices and rural hospitals did not receive their fair share. The Trump Administration compounded the dilemma by firing the HHS Inspector General, Christi Grimm, who had worked in the OIG office since 1999.

Goozner concludes his editorial with a telling quote from Warren Buffet. Talking about recessions, Buffet likes to say, *"Only when the tide goes out do you discover who's been swimming naked."* Goozner's conclusion: *"Healthcare's tide is out. Everyone is naked."*

TMR's Opinion - Goozner's right! The financing mechanisms for American healthcare are broken beyond easy repair. Unlike other developed nations, America stands alone in not providing universal healthcare to all its citizens. **TMR** supports the Eichhorn-Hutchinson comprehensive universal healthcare plan whose design addresses the critical flaws exposed by the pandemic. Based on Germany's approach that provides seamless coverage through employment and the government, the E-H plan provides choice along with a public option, and reduces administrative waste, drug costs and medically related bankruptcies. It is described in detail in "Healing American Healthcare: A Plan to Provide Quality Care to All While Saving $1 Trillion a Year," available from Amazon or Barnes & Noble.

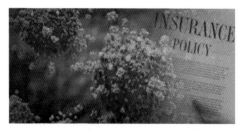

Some Workers Face Looming Cutoffs in Health Insurance, by Reed Abelson, New York Times, 9/28/20

TMR Topline™ - Many businesses have tried to keep their workers insured during the pandemic, relying on government aid, including the Paycheck Protection Program, to pay for premiums through the spring and summer. In addition to laying off workers (13.6 million unemployed), businesses are cutting expenses like health coverage. An analysis from Avalere Health estimates that 12 million will lose employer-sponsored health insurance (ESI) by year end, including 2 million Black and 3 million Hispanic people. Stan Dorn, the director of the National Center for Coverage Innovation at Families USA, stated *"The odds are we are on track to have the largest coverage losses in our history."*

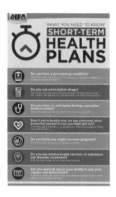

As COVID-19 Recession Extended Into Summer 2020, More Than 3 Million Lost Employer-Sponsored Health Insurance Coverage and 2 Million Became Uninsured, by A. Gangopadhyaya, M. Karpman and J. Aarons, Urban Institute, 9/17/20

TMR Topline™ - The Household Pulse Survey offers a snapshot of how health insurance coverage changed between April 23–May 12 and July 9–21, 2020. Through mid-July, 5.2 million non-elderly adults lost ESI. Younger adults, men and adults who did not attend college made up the majority of ESI losses. Hispanic adults were disproportionately represented.

Short-term plans spent little on medical claims in 2019, by Shelby Livingston, Modern Healthcare, 9/28/20

TMR Topline™ - According to the latest data from the National Association of Insurance Commissioners (NAIC), short-term insurance plans spent roughly 62 cents of every dollar they collected in premiums on members' medical claims in 2019. Short-term health plans don't have to cover preexisting health conditions or the ACA's 10 essential health benefits. The ACA requires that large health insurers spend at least 85 cents of every premium dollar on medical claims or rebate the difference to subscribers (i.e., a Medical Loss Ratio, or MLR, of 85%).

A June report from the House Energy and Commerce Committee estimated that 3 million people are enrolled in such plans. The plans often exclude conditions including diabetes, cancer, heart disease, arthritis, substance use and mental health disorders. Chair Frank Pallone (D-N.J.) stated *"These plans are a bad deal for consumers and oftentimes leave patients saddled with thousands of dollars in medical debt."*

TMR's Take - U.S. Census Bureau data for 2019 estimates that 92% of Americans (293.5 million) had health insurance while 8% (26.1 million) were uninsured. ESI accounted for 183 million of the insured population, Medicare 58.8 million, Medicaid 55.9 million and individual plans 33.2 million. While 220.6 million Americans had some form of private health insurance coverage in 2019, that is dropping in 2020. While some of those losing coverage will qualify for Medicaid, most will join the ranks of the uninsured. Administered by private sector contractors, the Medicare program's MLR is 97%. More on that in the next issue of **TMR.**

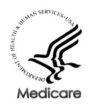

Medicare Beneficiaries Require More Financial, Coverage Support, by Karen Davis and Amber Willink The Commonwealth Fund, 9/23/20

TMR Topline™ - The Commonwealth Fund conducted a study to learn more about care affordability for low-income Medicare beneficiaries during the Covid-19 pandemic. Traditional Medicare's benefit design has coverage gaps that can leave beneficiaries financially vulnerable. Roughly 28% (17 million) have incomes below 150% of the federal poverty level ($18,000/ year for a single person). Many had been in the workforce, lost jobs and will have difficulty regaining employment. One-third spend more than 20% of income on premiums and medical care.

Congress enacted measures to support health care providers, but more needs to be done to help low-income Medicare beneficiaries without supplemental coverage. Policy changes to be considered include waiving cost-sharing for beneficiaries with Covid-19, offering Medicare as a choice for those ages 55 to 64, expanding benefits to include preventive and maintenance dental, vision, and hearing services and capping out-of-pocket costs.

Should Medicare adapt these changes, new measures would have to be developed to ensure the solvency of the Medicare Part A trust fund. The researchers concluded: *"Although Medicare provides a stable, trusted source of health insurance for older adults and younger people with disabilities, the program's benefit design can leave beneficiaries exposed to high out-of-pocket costs and premiums. In the current crisis, this is particularly a concern for those without supplemental coverage. "*

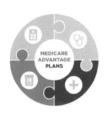

Medicare Advantage insurers plan for bigger footprints, more telehealth by Shelby Livingston Modern Healthcare 10/1/20

TMR Topline™ - More than 3.2 million seniors will become eligible for Medicare by the beginning of 2021 and Medicare Advantage (MA) insurers are expanding their service areas and adding new benefits to compete for members in this fast-growing market. UnitedHealthcare plans to sell coverage in four additional states and 300 new counties. Cigna is adding 67 new counties to its service area. Aetna and Humana also announced plans to reach more seniors. Eyeing this market potential, Walmart has joined with Clover Health to offer MA plans in several counties in Georgia.

MA plans are the fastest growing segment of the health insurance market. The federal government expects MA enrollment to grow by 10% in 2021 to 26.9 million, with 4 in 10 Medicare beneficiaries getting coverage from an MA plan. Ten years ago, only 25%, or about 11 million, had MA coverage. MA plans must cover all the benefits included in traditional Medicare but can offer additional benefits including dental and vision coverage. The Trump administration has added more flexibility to MA plans, allowing them to offer additional benefits such as home-delivered meals and transportation.

Most MA insurers are offering more telehealth benefits. Doctors and patients have turned to virtual care during the Covid-19 pandemic. CMS estimates that more than 94% of MA plans will offer telehealth benefits next year, up from 58% of plans in 2020. Some insurers include behavioral health visits and virtual physical therapy as telehealth services. There will be 4,800 plans in the MA market for 2021, averaging 47 plans per county, up from 39 this year. Individuals with end-stage kidney disease will also be able to purchase plans for the first time.

TMR's Take - These articles contrast the plight of 17 million low-income Medicare beneficiaries with the choices available to more affluent beneficiaries in MA plans. The first October issue described the turmoil in the commercial insurance market as millions lost employer-sponsored coverage and the inadequacy of short-term plans. Access to affordable healthcare for all Americans continues to be a critical issue. To be continued.

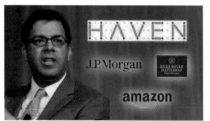

Why Jeff Bezos, Warren Buffett, and Jamie Dimon gave up on their venture to disrupt US healthcare, by Annalisa Merelli, Quartz, 1/6/21

TMR Topline™ - Three years ago the media were speculating that the combined might of Amazon, Berkshire-Hathaway and JPMorgan Chase would disrupt the U.S.'s muddle of a medical system. The companies employ a combined 1.2 million people spread around the country. Surgeon and author (The Checklist Manifesto) Dr. Atul Gawande's installation as CEO would guarantee the success of not-for-profit Haven. So why did Haven fail? Among the reasons detailed in the article: Haven had a mission, but never quite a strategy. Its goal, *"create simpler, high-quality healthcare at lower costs,"* was a vision with no business plan. Another problem was the divergence of interests among the three companies. Jeff Becker, an analyst at Forrester said, *"Haven is yet another cautionary tale to outsiders that hope to disrupt the industry that their ambition is likely unrealistic and that solving key industry problems proves to be far more difficult than most anticipate."* Healthcare's complicated.

Types of Headaches

Not enough time, not enough clarity: Payers push back on CMS prior authorization rule, by Rebecca Fifer, HEALTHCAREDIVE, 1/6/21

TMR Topline™ - First proposed in mid-December, HHS's attempt to streamline the prior authorization process is meeting fierce resistance from payers. It's part of the Trump administration's push to improve the electronic exchange of health data between payers, providers, and patients, and builds off the massive interoperability regulations finalized in March. If finalized, the rule would require payers to build and maintain standardized application programming interfaces (APIs), technology that allows different computer systems to send and receive information, for payer-to-provider and payer-to-patient sharing of health data, including prior authorization data.

America's Health Insurance Plans (AHIP) contends that it is *"distracting from the crucial fight against the pandemic as we enter a key phase in defeating Covid-19."* The proposed rule excludes Medicare Advantage plans.

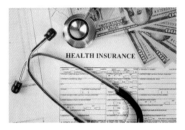

Lavish bonus? Luxury trip? Health benefits brokers will have to disclose what they receive from the insurance industry, by Marshall Allen, ProPublica, 1/6/21

TMR Topline™ - Buried in the coronavirus relief package is a requirement that health benefit brokers disclose to employers how much they make from insurance carriers. ProPublica showed in 2019 how the insurance industry influences the consultants behind the scenes with cash and gifts—from six-figure bonuses to swanky island getaways. A broker's base commission can range from 3-6% of the total premiums. Employer sponsored health plans cover about 150 million Americans. Michael Thompson, president of the National Alliance of Healthcare Purchaser Coalitions, which represents employers, called the new disclosure requirements an encouraging *"step in the right direction."*

TMR's Take - Haven's failure to gain traction despite a base of 1.2 million employees results from the absurd complexity of America's fragmented healthcare system. It was unable to develop the critical mass needed to gain economies of scale. **TMR** supports HHS's attempt to streamline payers use of prior authorizations and would go even further, eliminating the procedure altogether. Countries with universal healthcare rely on post-treatment review to identify abuses. Payers continued use of this tactic to delay, defer, and deny care second-guesses medical judgment and adds cost with little or no benefit. Likewise, the need for employers to use brokers contributes to the U.S.'s high healthcare costs.

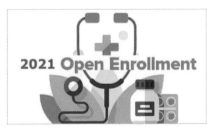

Biden Extends Health Insurance Marketplace Through Summer, by Chelsea Cirruzzo, U.S. News, 3/23/21

TMR Topline™ - The Biden administration has extended the exchange special enrollment period to August 15, giving consumers in 36 states three more months to sign up for coverage through HealthCare.gov. The change will allow more people to take advantage of greater financial assistance for marketplace plans under the American Rescue Plan Act.

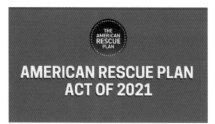

Will the American Rescue Plan Reduce the Number of Uninsured Americans?, by Sara R. Collins and Gabriella Aboulafia, The Commonwealth Fund, 3/22/21

TMR Topline™ - The American Rescue Plan Act (ARPA) contains the most extensive health insurance improvements for Americans since enactment of the ACA 11 years ago. With 30 million uninsured, the Commonwealth Fund looked at who the uninsured are and how the ARPA will help get them covered. 14.9 million are eligible for subsidized marketplace plans or may have an offer of employer coverage. HHS estimates that 11.2 million uninsured people had incomes that made them eligible for subsidized coverage through the marketplaces and 3.6 million had incomes too high to qualify for these subsidies. Another 6.4 million are eligible for Medicaid or the Children's Health Insurance Program (CHIP) but are not enrolled. 4.8 million have incomes below the poverty level and live in Medicaid non-expansion states. They are not eligible for marketplace plan subsidies but may be eligible for their existing state Medicaid program. Finally, 3.1 million are undocumented immigrants who are not allowed to enroll under either option.

The Congressional Budget Office estimates that 2.5 million will get coverage through the increased financial support in the ARPA. The authors also offer several additional policy changes that are needed to help get more people covered. These include making the ARPA premium tax credit enhancements permanent, improving the cost-protection of marketplace plans and allowing people with incomes below poverty in Medicaid non-expansion states to enroll in marketplace plans.

TMR's Take - This Commonwealth Fund's data suggest that with ARPA's enactment nearly 90% of uninsured Americans are potentially eligible for health insurance coverage. The Biden administration needs to take this message to the American public, especially in states that did not expand Medicaid. The CBO's estimate was done prior to the extension of the open enrollment period. With effective messaging, the number could be much higher.

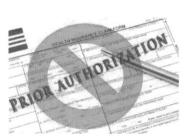

Doctors say prior authorization led to life-threatening delays in care, by Matti Gellman, Modern Healthcare, 4/7/21

TMR Topline™ - A recent AMA survey found that slow prior authorization (PA) protocols contributed to care delivery delays and poor treatment outcomes for some patients during the surge in Covid-19 cases last winter. Nearly all physicians surveyed said they spent about 16 hours weekly seeking an average of 40 PAs for patient care. One-third of physicians reportedly had a patient suffer a serious medical event because of delayed access to treatment and 90% said PA had a negative impact on a patient's treatment outcome.

Although health plans claim that their processes are informed by evidence-based medicine, one-third of physicians disagreed. AMA President Dr. Susan R. Bailey said, *"This hard-learned lesson must guide a re-examination of administrative burdens imposed by health insurers, often without any justification,"* calling for increased transparency in insurers' PA criteria and the streamlining of low-value prior authorization requirements.

Payment is due when services are rendered

When money talks. Why cash pay is becoming more popular, by Nona Tepper, Modern Healthcare, 4/13/21

TMR Topline™ - Sidecar Health founder Patrick Quigley's *"aha"* moment came after an MRI exam when he was left with a $1,300 bill after insurance. A few months later, needing an MRI at the same facility, he offered to pay with his debit card rather than deal with his high-deductible health plan. The cash price was just $330. A 2019 study by Vanderbilt University found that providers will cut their prices by up to 40% for patients who pay with cash.

The Covid-19 pandemic is forcing health systems to be more flexible in how services are paid for in response to changing consumer expectations. Sidecar Health is one of many startups (e.g., CashMD, Medibid, Bind) targeting millennial and Gen Z customers while leaving complex and chronic condition management to more experienced players. Several studies show that providers spend 40% of their time dealing with administrative processes that distract from patient care. Sidecar aims to expand coverage to the 15 million uninsured or underinsured, offering to reimburse consumers for the average price of their service in their market. It surveyed 120,000 doctors in 10 practice areas to create a predictive pricing algorithm that determines the cash price for 170,000 different services anywhere in the U.S. It will offer its first employer-sponsored plan next year and will eventually follow other start-ups into the lucrative Medicare market.

TMR's Take - Both articles illustrate the administrative waste so prevalent in U.S. healthcare. More disturbing is the potential for patient harm from insurer-driven delays.

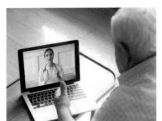

Prospective CMS Administrators confirmation hearing highlights Congress's desire to expand telehealth coverage, by Nick Hut, HFMA, 4/21/21

TMR Topline™ - In the confirmation hearing for Chiquita Brooks-LaSure, the nominee for CMS administrator, it became clear that telehealth will be a key part of Medicare and Medicaid policy. Said Sen. Ron Wyden (D-Ore.), chairman of the Finance Committee, *"As a result of the pandemic, we've removed some of the roadblocks for people to actually get to a telehealth provider. We're going to have to make those kinds of changes permanent in addition to working on the critical reimbursement issue."*

Other Committee members echoed Wyden's comments, noting that it is an area of potential bipartisan agreement. Other policy areas discussed during the hearing included surprise billing, prescription drug pricing and the impact of deferred care caused by the pandemic. Sen. Robert Menendez (D-N.J.) cited a study showing primary care visits declined by 21% in Q2 2020 compared with the previous two years.

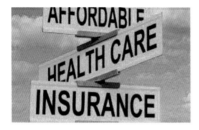

Affordable Health Care Is Fundamental to Families' Economic Security, by Sara Collins, The Commonwealth Fund, 4/28/21

TMR Topline™ - Nearly 1 million people have enrolled in health insurance coverage through the Affordable Care Act's (ACA's) marketplaces since the Biden administration reopened them in February. Enactment of the American Rescue Plan (ARP) means many of these new enrollees, as well as the 12 million who were already enrolled in private insurance through the ACA, are paying much less or had their premiums reduced to zero based on the law's temporary premium subsidies. Collins suggests three policy changes that would build on the success of the ARP subsidies to improve coverage and provide permanent financial relief to many families:

1. As the American Families Plan proposes, make the temporary ARP marketplace subsidies permanent. The Urban Institute estimates that this would reduce the number of uninsured by 4.2 million in 2022.

2. Opening the ACA marketplaces to the uninsured in the 14 states that have not expanded Medicaid would provide an estimated 2 million uninsured people with an immediate coverage option.

3. Capping employee cost sharing in employer plans at 8.5% of income would mean that no one would have to spend more than that on health insurance.

The Biden administration and Congress have moved to provide economic security for low- and middle-income families. The data clearly suggests that without affordable health care, no family can be economically secure.

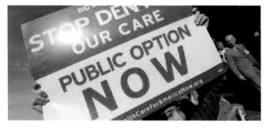

Effective public option would need to cut provider rates, expert says, by Jessie Hellman, Modern Healthcare, 5/6/21

TMR Topline™ - Matthew Fiedler, a fellow in economic studies at the USC-Brookings Schaeffer Initiative for Health Policy has published an analysis that suggests a public option having lower premiums than private plans that saves consumers money would need to pay providers less. The public option would need to set provider rates—like Medicare does—and require provider participation. *"The main way a public option could reduce premiums is by paying providers less,"* Fiedler said. *"It's absolutely true that paying providers less is politically controversial."*

In recent years as ideas like the public option and Medicare for All have gained traction, provider and insurance groups have increased their lobbying efforts opposing these proposals. Hospital groups argue that Medicare rates are too low and a public option would just expand this pay structure that they believe is unfair. However, the Medicare Payment Advisory Commission (MEDPAC) estimates Medicare's prices exceeded providers' cost of care by 8% in 2019.

A brief released this week by the Center for American Progress (CAP) also concluded that a key element of a public option's success is lowering provider payment rates, especially for hospitals. Maura Calsyn, managing director of health policy at CAP said *"It's not just lowering hospital prices or lowering prices in a way that is not thoughtful. The idea really is to rethink how those dollars on reimbursement are spent."* The CAP brief proposed that a public option would improve health equity by expanding access to care for the underserved by lowering costs and reinvesting savings back into those communities without damaging struggling providers and hospitals.

TMR's Take - Access to healthcare is a fundamental human right, not a privilege for those who can afford it. Powerful lobbies already are lined up to oppose these changes that would benefit ordinary Americans.

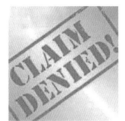

Looming UnitedHealthcare policy on coverage of emergency department care draws opposition from hospitals, physicians, by Nick Hut, HFMA, 6/9/21

TMR Topline™ - UnitedHealthcare (UHC), the nation's leading commercial health insurer by market share, announced a new policy directed at denying ED claims it deems nonemergent. UHC will assess such claims based on the patient's presenting problem, the intensity of services performed and other patient complication factors and external causes, with an estimated 10% denial rate. To reverse the denial, the hospital must submit an attestation that the patient's visit met the prudent layperson standard for an emergency. *"If the attestation is submitted within the required time frame, the claim will typically be processed according to the plan's emergency benefits,"* UHC wrote in its post about the coverage policy.

The American Hospital Association (AHA) and American College of Emergency Physicians (ACEP) each is petitioning UHC to reverse the policy. ACEP cited CDC statistics showing that only 3% of ED visits are nonurgent. ACEP President Mark Rosenberg, DO, MBA, said UHC is *"expecting patients to self-diagnose a potential medical emergency before seeing a physician, and then punishing them financially if they are incorrect."* A UHC official said that if a member goes to the ED with chest pain and receives a final diagnosis of heartburn, the visit would be covered once the provider attests that the case met the prudent layperson standard.

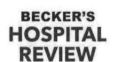

UnitedHealthcare must permanently rescind ER policy, hospitals demand, by Morgan Haefner, Becker's Hospital Review, 6/11/21

TMR Topline™ - Although UnitedHeathcare (UHC) has paused its controversial policy to deny ED claims it deems nonemergent until the end of the public health emergency, both the American Hospital Association and the Federation of American Hospitals have called for it to be permanently rescinded.

TMR's Take - Hospitals are appropriately outraged by UHC's arbitrary policy, especially given evidence that patients are using alternatives to ED visits. Dr. Rosenberg knows whereof he speaks. As chief of emergency medicine at St. Joseph's Health in Paterson, NJ, he's responsible for the 4th busiest ED in the country. UHC is all about profit, not service to its members, proving again the adage: *"For-profit enterprises operate to benefit their stockholders; not-for-profit enterprises operate to benefit their stakeholders."* The U.S. should emulate France and Germany where health insurers are not-for-profit but compete fiercely for business based on service to their members.

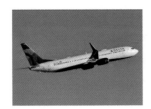

Delta Air Lines health surcharge for vaccines could cascade across industries, by Eleanor Mueller, Oriana Pawlyk and Tatiana Monnay, Politico, 8/25/2021

TMR Topline™ - In a memo to all employees, Delta Airlines CEO Ed Bastian served notice of a $200/month health insurance surcharge for unvaccinated Delta employees to offset medical costs from a coronavirus infection. Delta said the average hospital stay for Covid has cost the airline $50,000 per person, noting *"This surcharge will be necessary to address the financial risk the decision to not vaccinate is creating for our company."* The Airline Pilots Association voiced concerns about the surcharge, saying that Delta needs to *"bargain with the Delta MEC over any employer-mandated vaccination for pilots."* To date, over 75% of Delta employees have been vaccinated.

TMR Take – The carrot didn't work, but the stick might. The rapid response by public and private organizations to impose vaccine mandates based on the FDA approval may finally move America closer to herd immunity.

CHAPTER 7

Big Pharma: Miracle Drugs at Sky High Prices

T HE HIGH COSTS OF BRAND NAME DRUGS HAVE BEEN A FRONT-BURNER ISSUE FOR AMERICANS, ESPECIALLY Medicare beneficiaries, for years. In the 2016 Presidential campaign both candidates promised action on prescription drug pricing. The Democratic candidate, Hillary Clinton, advocated for universal and affordable quality healthcare for all Americans, promising to:

- Bring down out-of-pocket costs,
- Reduce the cost of prescription drugs,
- Protect consumers from unjustified prescription drug price increases, and
- Incentivize states to expand Medicaid.

The Republican candidate, Donald Trump, wanted Congress to act to:

- Completely repeal Obamacare,
- Allow sale of health insurance across state lines,
- Remove barriers to entry into free markets for drug providers that offer safe, reliable and cheaper products, and
- Block-grant Medicaid to the states.

Five years later, little has changed, and the cost of brand name drugs continue to increase at a rate far higher than inflation, and now represent 10% of America's healthcare costs. According to Statista, U.S. prescription drug spending was $358.7 billion in 2020. In June, the FDA approved Biogen's Aduhelm for treatment of Alzheimer's disease despite mixed clinical trial results. Priced at $56,000/year, if only one million of the six million Americans with Alzheimer's were prescribed the drug, Medicare costs could exceed $50 billion annually. An independent analysis has suggested that $3,000-$8,400 would be a reasonable price range for Aduhelm.

On a less negative note, in July the FDA approved Viatris Inc.'s Semglee as the first biosimilar to substitute for Lantus, a widely used fast-acting insulin. A month's supply of Semglee injector pens will cost about $150-190, about 40% of the cost of a month's supply of Lantus. Insulin was first discovered in 1921 by three researchers at the University of Toronto. They sold the original patent to the University of Toronto for $1, believing that a drug this important should always be available and affordable to individuals who needed it. They were rewarded with the Nobel Prize, but none of the billions in profits that the pharmaceutical industry gleaned from their discovery.

Over the course of the past 100 years, pharmaceutical industry's drug discoveries have been a major contributor to increasing life expectancy – and to incredible profit margins for those companies. The Pharmaceutical Research and Manufacturers of America (PhRMA) has become one of the most powerful lobbyists in Washington. The industry employs over 880 full-time lobbyists whose job is to educate and influence elected officials and key government employees. It also supports Political Action Committees (PACs) to push forward the industry's legislative interests.

Eighteen months into the worst global pandemic in more than a century, how do U.S. drug costs compare with other countries? Studies by both the Commonwealth Fund and the Harvard School of Public Health indicate that Americans use about the same pharmaceuticals in roughly the same amounts on a per capita basis as other developed countries do. The same international pharmaceutical companies develop, produce and market them, but in 2018 the prices Americans paid were 2.56 times higher than the average in 32 other OECD member nations according to a RAND Corporation analysis. Total drug spending for the 32 countries was $795 billion and the U.K., France and Italy had the lowest prescription drug prices among the G-7 nations.

What makes them different? The other countries in these studies all have national health care systems that negotiate the prices for drug therapies for their residents. The Medicare Modernization Act of 2003 provided partial prescription drug coverage for Medicare beneficiaries but with significant limitations due to the influence of PhRMA (and the insurance lobby). It required Medicare to pay list price for drugs, leaving the door wide open for insurers to develop Medicare Advantage (MA) plans to compete with Medicare. MA plans can negotiate drug prices; Medicare cannot.

The 32 articles summarized in this chapter include several that track the success of Operation Warp Speed's accelerated development of safe and effective vaccines for Covid-19. With much of the fundamental research done in government labs following the 2003 SARS outbreak, both the Pfizer/BioNTech and Moderna mRNA vaccines received emergency use authorizations from the FDA in December 2020. This breakthrough technology is the 21st century equivalent of the Salk and Sabin vaccines that conquered polio in the 1950s.

Unfortunately, many of the articles summarized in this chapter reported on litigation against and settlements with major drug companies for a variety of abuses.

Pharmaceutical Three Minute Reads

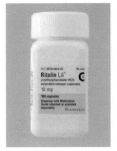

U.S. states accuse 26 drug makers of generic drug price fixing in sweeping lawsuit, by Diane Bartz and Jonathan Stempel, Reuters, 6/10/20

TMR Topline™ - The Connecticut Attorney General and 50 other states and territories filed suit against 26 drug manufacturers accusing them of conspiring to reduce competition and drive-up generic drug prices. From 2009-2016, the suit alleges that Novartis, Teva, Mylan, Pfizer and others rigged the market for more than 80 drugs including Ritalin, Xalatan, Differin, Dilantin, and Lotrimin AF Cream. Noting that generic pharmaceutical executives were in constant communication colluding to fix prices and restrain competition, Connecticut Attorney General William Tong said *"They took steps to evade accountability."*

TMR's Take - If the allegations ultimately are proven, the companies' conduct is the antithesis of the capitalist free enterprise system. Diabetic Americans are familiar with Sanofi and Novo Nordisk's high insulin prices. Generic drugs are supposed to be affordable.

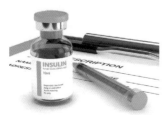

Pharmaceutical industry sues to block Minnesota insulin law, Associated Press, 7/1/20

TMR Topline™ - The Pharmaceutical Research and Manufacturers of America (PhRMA) is suing to overturn a Minnesota law that that requires them to provide emergency and longer-term insulin supplies to diabetics who can't afford them, alleging that violates the takings clause of the Constitution's Fifth Amendment. The Act is named for Alex Smith, a 26-year-old Minneapolis man who had aged off his mother's insurance and couldn't afford the $1,300 per month cost of the drug and test supplies. He died in 2017 of complications from rationing his insulin. PhRMA blames health plans and pharmacy benefit managers for insulin's high costs.

TMR's Take - When Dr. Banting and his colleagues discovered insulin in 1923, they sold their patent for $1 to the University of Toronto because they wanted everyone who needed their medication to be able to afford it. The U.S. is 15% of the global insulin market but produces nearly half of the industry's insulin revenues. "The absurdly high cost of insulin, explained" provides a deeper dive into the insulin pricing controversy.

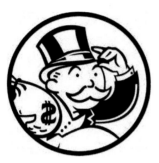

Novartis pays $678M to resolve suit over sham doctor outings, Associated Press, 7/1/20

TMR Topline™ - Acting Manhattan U.S. Attorney Audrey Strauss announced that Novartis Pharmaceutical Corp. will pay $678 million to the U.S. government and various states to settle a 2011 whistleblower lawsuit over a sham speaker program. The company admitted giving doctors cash, golf and fishing trips, and lavish meals to induce them to prescribe Novartis cardiovascular and diabetes drugs. William F. Sweeney Jr., head of New York's FBI office, called the company's conduct *"reprehensible and dishonest,"* noting that *"Greed replaced the responsibility the public expects from those who practice medicine."*

TMR's Take - Greed is not good. Novartis joins a long list of drug companies including Eli Lilly, Merck, Pfizer, Amgen, Johnson & Johnson and Abbott who have reached settlements for violating the False Claims Act and Anti-Kickback Statutes.

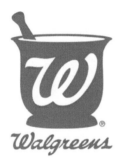

Walgreens Boots Alliance invests $1B in VillageMD to open 500+ medical clinics, by Laura Dyrda, Beckers Hospital Review, 7/8/2020

TMR Topline™ - VillageMD, a primary care startup that focuses on helping manage chronic care conditions, partnered with Walgreens at five co-located clinics in the Houston area. The stores have reported high patient satisfaction and increased medication adherence. The $1 billion investment will enable VillageMD to open 500-700 more clinics, half in areas with shortages of medical professionals. It already manages over 1,000 clinics in nine states.

TMR's Take - Americans trust their pharmacists. Rival CVS Health is opening HealthHubs in its stores to help customers better manage their health. With the looming physician shortage, will there be doctors to staff them?

Trump signs series of executive orders aimed at lowering drug costs, by Noah Higgins, Jasmine Kim, Berkeley Lovelace, Jr., CNBC, 7/27/20

TMR Topline™ - On Friday, July 24, President Trump signed four executive orders aimed at lowering the high cost of prescription drugs, an estimated $335 billion in 2018. The orders:

1. Require community health centers to pass the discounts they receive on insulin and EpiPens directly to patients.

2. Allow states, pharmacies, and wholesalers to import drugs from Canada.

3. Prevent pharmacy benefit managers from retaining all the discounts that they receive from manufacturers; and

4. Allow Medicare to implement an international pricing index to bring drug prices in line with what other nations pay.

Although he signed the fourth order, President Trump was holding it until Aug. 24 to give the industry time to *"come up with something"* to reduce drug prices. Health and Human Services Secretary Alex Azar stated that drug companies currently pay about $150 billion in undisclosed kickbacks to middlemen and that the executive orders, when implemented, would save seniors about $30 billion a year. Predictably, the Pharmaceutical Research and Manufacturers of America (PhRMA), called them a *"reckless distraction"* to the COVID-19 pandemic and a step towards socialized health care.

TMR's Take - The 2016 Republican platform pledged to *"Remove barriers to entry into free markets for drug providers that offer safe, reliable and cheaper products."* The second executive order is a step in that direction. It will take several months for implementing regulations to be drafted, commented on, finalized, and issued.

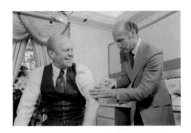

Gerald Ford Rushed Out a Vaccine. It was a Fiasco, by Rick Perlstein, The New York Times, 9/2/2020

TMR Topline™ - President Trump is considering an *"emergency use authorization"* for a Covid-19 vaccine before Phase 3 clinical trials are completed. The CDC has instructed the states to be ready to distribute a vaccine by November 1. History suggests that rushing out a vaccine before it has been vetted as safe and effective is a risky gamble.

An early 1976 outbreak of a new strain of the H1N1 swine flu virus at Fort Dix prompted the Ford administration to fast track a vaccine to prevent an epidemic. The vaccine was released in the fall and 45 million Americans were vaccinated. Side effects: 450 developed Guillain-Barre syndrome; more than 30 died. The vaccination program was cancelled. One soldier died from the swine flu.

TMR's Take - How much risk are Americans willing to take? The anti-vaxxers will have a field day opposing a vaccine that has not been proven to be safe and effective. It's a risky gamble that could do more harm than good.

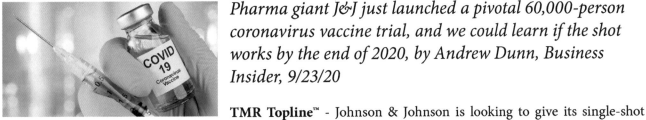

Pharma giant J&J just launched a pivotal 60,000-person coronavirus vaccine trial, and we could learn if the shot works by the end of 2020, by Andrew Dunn, Business Insider, 9/23/20

TMR Topline™ - Johnson & Johnson is looking to give its single-shot vaccine to 60,000 volunteers around the world, becoming the fourth US backed program to begin phase three clinical trials. The other experimental shots being tested are two-dose regimens, with injections given a few weeks apart. Dr. Anthony Fauci said results from J&J's trial will likely lag a month or two behind studies that started in July or August, like Moderna's and Pfizer's. J&J's chief scientist, Paul Stoffels, echoed Fauci's timeline: *"We hope to see an endpoint around the end of year or early next year."*

TMR's Take - Operation Warp Speed has already spent over $10 billion to fast-track Covid-19 vaccine development, helping vaccine makers to build out production capacity before knowing whether their vaccine is safe and effective. Hopes remain high that the investment will produce positive returns.

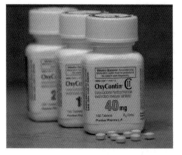

OxyContin maker Purdue Pharma pleads guilty in criminal case, by Geoff Mulvihill, Associated Press, 11/24/20

TMR Topline™ - Taking responsibility for its part in an opioid epidemic that has taken more than 470,000 lives over the past two decades, Purdue Pharma pleaded guilty to three criminal charges, admitting to: 1. Impeding the DEA's efforts to combat the addiction crisis; 2. Not maintaining an effective program to prevent drugs from being diverted to the black market; 3. paying doctors through a speakers program to induce them to write more prescriptions for its painkillers; and 4. paying an electronic medical records company to send doctors information on patients that encouraged them to prescribe opioids.

The pleas were part of a criminal and civil settlement with the Justice Department that includes $8.3 billion in forfeitures and penalties. The attorneys general for about half the states opposed the federal settlement, as well as the company's proposed settlement in bankruptcy court. Critics also want to see individuals held accountable.

The wealthy Sackler family agreed to give up control and pay $225 million to the federal government to settle civil claims, but no criminal charges have yet been filed. Internal Purdue documents obtained as part of the investigation show family members pushing for OxyContin sales even as opioid-related deaths rose.

TMR's Take - The proposed settlement tops Purdue's $601 million 2007 settlement for off label promotion of Oxycontin, joining Glaxo Smith Kline, Pfizer, Abbott and Eli Lilly in the billion-dollar settlement club.

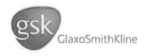

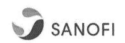

GSK/Sanofi Covid vaccine delayed until end of next year, by Ian Sample, Science Editor, The Guardian, 12/11/20

TMR Topline™ - After interim results from a phase 1/2 trial revealed that it failed to produce a strong immune response in older people, GlaxoSmithKline and its French partner, Sanofi, decided to reformulate the vaccine and launch another phase 2 trial in February with an aim to deliver approved shots in the last quarter of 2021, barring any further setbacks. The setback is a reminder of the difficulty of developing a safe, effective vaccine.

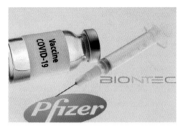

Some vaccine doses kept too cold, Pfizer having manufacturing issues, U.S. officials say, by Carl O'Donnell, Rebecca Spaulding, Reuters, 12/16/20

TMR Topline™ - The Pfizer/BioNTech vaccine rollout has encountered some speed bumps. At least two trays of doses delivered in California needed to be replaced after their storage temperatures dipped below -80C. Officials are investigating whether storing the vaccines at temperatures below -70C poses a safety or efficacy risk. Pfizer also has reported some production issues and CEO Alfred Bourla is asking the U.S. government to use the Defense Production Act to relieve some *"critical supply limitations."* UPS and FedEx are developing contingency plans for vaccine deliveries given forecasts of severe winter weather in some parts of the U.S.

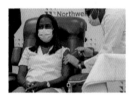

When will other coronavirus vaccines in the pipeline come to N.J.?, by Karin Price Mueller, Star-Ledger, 12/16/20

TMR Topline™ - With the Pfizer vaccine now in use and Moderna's vaccine recently approved, the writer provided an update on three others in the pipeline.

Johnson & Johnson – J&J's vaccine is currently in a Phase 3 study using some 42,000 participants. Its vaccine contains the adenovirus and only requires one dose. It uses genetic material from Covid-19 that should cause the immune system to create antibodies against it. First results from the trial are expected in January.

AstraZeneca - Its two-dose vaccine also uses an adenovirus, has completed Phase 3 clinical trials on 20,000 people, and deemed safe and effective by an independent scientific analysis published last week in The Lancet. While a standard two-dose regime was 62% effective, when people received a low dose followed by a standard dose it was 90% effective.

Merck - Merck CEO Kenneth Frazier stated that its work is *"not nearly as advanced"* as Pfizer and Moderna, but its antiviral has moved into Phase 3 trials.

TMR's Take - With both the Pfizer/BioNTech and Moderna vaccines receiving EUA approval from the FDA, and others far along in the pipeline, there's a light at the end of the tunnel as this pandemic year ends. The New York Times Coronavirus Vaccine Tracker reports 63 vaccines in clinical trials on humans with 18 in the final stages of testing. Nonetheless, challenges remain. **TMR** hopes that 2021 will bring a return to a new normal by mid-year. **Have a safe and healthy holiday season!**

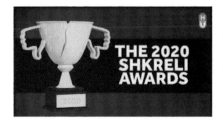

'Shkreli Awards' Shame Healthcare Profiteers, by Cheryl Clark, Contributing Writer, MedPage Today 1/6/21

TMR Topline™ - Named for entrepreneur Martin Shkreli, who gained notoriety in 2015 by raising the price of Daraprim (the only known cure for toxoplasmosis) from $13.50 to $750 a pill, the Lown Institute's 2020 Annual Shkreli Awards focus on *"pandemic profiteers."* Here are the top three of the ten awards:

- **3rd Place** - four California hospital systems that refused to take Covid-19 patients or delayed transfers from hospitals that were out of beds. A *Wall Street Journal* investigation found the refusals or delays were based on patients' ability to pay; many were on Medicaid or uninsured.
- **2nd Place** - vaccine maker Moderna, which set a price of $32-37 per dose, more than the U.S. agreed to pay for other Covid vaccines. Moderna received $955 million in federal funding to develop its vaccine working in partnership with scientists at the National Institutes of Health.
- **1st Place** – Jared Kushner and the federal government's Project Airbridge, to *"airlift PPE from overseas and bring it to the U.S. quickly"* to go to designated pandemic hotspots. Instead, the supplies were given to six private medical supply companies to sell to the highest bidder, setting off a bidding war among the states. No officials from the 10 hardest hit counties said that they received PPE from Project Airbridge.

TMR's Take –Wallet biopsies during a pandemic? EMTALA was enacted in 1986 to end them. Moderna's pricing seems direct from the Gordon Gekko *"Greed is good"* school in 1987's *"Wall Street."* But TMR agrees. The Project Airbridge fiasco tops them all.

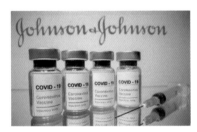

Johnson & Johnson Applies For Emergency Use Authorization For COVID-19 Vaccine, by Dustin Jones, NPR, 2/4/21

TMR Topline™ - J&J has applied to the FDA for an emergency use authorization for its Janssen vaccine. If granted, J&J aims to supply 100 million doses in the first half of 2021. Overall, it is 66% effective in preventing moderate to severe Covid-19 four weeks after the shot is administered. J&J said the vaccine was 72% effective in the U.S., compared to 66% in Latin America and 57% in South Africa. Unlike Pfizer and Moderna, J&J's Janssen vaccine requires only one injection and can be stored for at least three months at 36-46F.

TMR's Take - Having a single dose vaccine available that does not require cold storage will, if approved by the FDA, accelerate getting more Americans vaccinated. Novovax is not far behind in the vaccine pipeline. Clinical trials of the two-dose vaccine are underway in the U.S. and Mexico. Like the J&J vaccine, it can be stored and shipped at normal refrigeration temperatures. If the trials are successful and the FDA approves, 110 million doses could be available by the end of June.

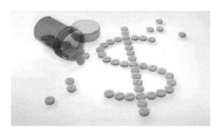

Here's How Much More the U.S. Spends on Rx Drugs, by Kristina Fiore, Director of Enterprise & Investigative Reporting, MedPage Today, 1/28/21

TMR Topline™ - On average, prescription drug prices were 2.56 times higher in the US than in 32 other OECD countries in 2018 according to a new RAND Corporation analysis. For brand name drugs, the U.S. paid an average of 3.44 times more, while generics cost slightly less - 84% of the price in other OECD nations. Generics also are prescribed more frequently in the U.S., accounting for 84% of volume compared with 35% of prescription drug volume in the other countries. Brand name drugs account for 82% of U.S. spending, but only 11% of volume."

The U.K., France, and Italy had the lowest prescription drug prices among the G-7 nations. Total drug spending for the 32 countries was $795 billion. RAND's Andrew Mulcahy, PhD, MPP commented *"Many of the most-expensive medications are the biologic treatments that we often see advertised on television,"* and expressed hope that competition from biosimilars will drive down prices and spending for biologics.

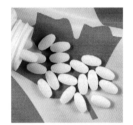

States Move Ahead With Canada Drug Importation While Awaiting Signal From Biden, by Phil Galewitz, Kaiser Health News, 1/29/21

TMR Topline™ - Florida, Colorado and several New England states are moving ahead with efforts to import prescription drugs from Canada, but it's not clear yet whether the Biden administration will allow states and the federal government to help Americans obtain lower-priced medications from Canada. PhRMA filed suit in D.C. federal court to stop the drug-purchasing initiatives in November. Prices are cheaper north of the border because Canada limits how much drugmakers can charge for medicines.

The 2003 Canadian drug importation law requires that the HHS Secretary certify that it could be done safely. HHS Secretary Alex Azar gave that approval in September, but HHS nominee Xavier Becerra's position is not known. Experts also question whether the savings could be significant given the expense of setting up and running an importation program given that some of the highest-priced drugs, such as insulin and other injectables, are excluded from drug importation.

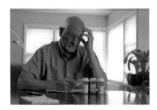

Seniors Face Crushing Drug Costs as Congress Stalls on Capping Medicare Out-Of-Pockets, by Harris Meyer, Kaiser Health News, 1/4/21

TMR Topline™ - KHN's series on drug pricing also covered the problems encountered by Medicare beneficiaries under Part D, particularly with cancer drugs. Except for very low-income beneficiaries, Part D drug plans have no cap on patients' 5% coinsurance costs once they hit $6,550 in drug spending. Medicare patients face modest out-of-pocket costs if their drugs are administered in the hospital or a doctor's office and they have a Medigap or Medicare Advantage plan, which cap those expenses. But during the past several years, dozens of effective drugs for cancer and other serious conditions have become available in oral form at the pharmacy. Medicare patients increasingly pay the Part D out-of-pocket costs with no set maximum.

According to a 2019 JAMA study, prices for 54 orally administered cancer drugs increased 40% from 2010 to 2018, averaging $167,904 for one year's treatment. The high drug prices and coverage gaps have forced many patients to rely on complicated financial assistance programs offered by drug companies and foundations. Fewer than 5% of U.S. cancer centers have experts on staff to help patients with problems paying for their care. A 2019 KFF survey found that nearly 70% of seniors want Congress to pass an annual limit on out-of-pocket drug spending for Medicare beneficiaries, but Congress cannot agree on how to fund such a limit.

TMR's Take - We've said it before: healthcare – it's *really* complicated! With so many middlemen involved in getting prescription drugs to the patient, it's little wonder that America's drug prices are the highest in the world. It's long past time to streamline and simplify the process.

From the Editor: The Biden Administration is tackling enormous challenges in its first 100 days, including its promise to continue on the path to universal healthcare by building on the ACA. One initiative with broad support is addressing the high cost of drugs in the U.S. "*Healing American Healthcare*" co-author and Coalition co-founder Ed Eichhorn shares his thoughts about moving forward with three plans that could reduce the high cost of drugs.

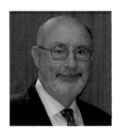

America Needs Lower Drug Prices Now – Here Are 3 Ways To Do It, The Healing American Healthcare Coalition Blog by Ed Eichhorn, 2/5/21

TMR Topline™ - The U.S. pays more than twice as much as the other 36 nation members of the OECD pay for prescription drugs. Studies of U.S. drug pricing and prescribing patterns have found that Americans use about the same amount of the same medications as do citizens of other OECD member nations. Americans just pay more for them. The other nations in the OECD negotiate drug prices on a national basis. America does not. Drug companies set their prices independently in the U.S. It will be difficult for lawmakers to develop legislation for a way to negotiate drug prices on a national basis even though this has worked in many other nations. There are three approaches that the U.S. could apply to bring down the cost of prescription drugs

Control Hospital Drug Pricing – Hospital markup of the drugs they administer to inpatients are not regulated. Hospitals should be limited to a 10% markup on any medication that they provide to their inpatients to cover their inventory costs.

Limit Orphan Drug Markups – The Orphan Drug Law was enacted in 1983. It encourages R&D to develop life-saving drugs for diseases that affect less than 200,000 people. It also provides a valuable incentive for drug companies to expand their businesses and to improve their profitability. The cost of these lifesaving medications has gone up by 64 times since 1983. This law should be amended to control the growth in orphan drug prices.

Allow Drug Importation – It is well known drugs are sold at lower prices in other countries. It makes sense to promote international ordering of drugs to lower costs for American consumers. Some states are beginning to negotiate with Canada to have the right to import drugs for their residents.

Applying these three approaches could go a long way towards lowering drug costs for all Americans.

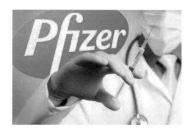

FDA panel says risks of Pfizer pain drug outweigh the benefits, by Damian Garde, STAT, 3/25/21

TMR Topline™ - A panel of expert advisors to the FDA voted 19-1 to reject Pfizer's application for approval of tanezumab, a non-addictive injectable painkiller, concluding that its risks might out-weigh its benefits. Developed to relieve osteoarthritis pain, it has been linked to rare but serious cases of joint damage. The 31 million Americans who suffer from osteoarthritis would welcome an alternative to opioids for pain relief. However, the FDA is unlikely to overrule its expert panel.

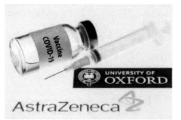

Fauci: AstraZeneca needs to 'straighten out' vaccine data, by Sarah Owermohle, Politico, 3/23/2021

TMR Topline™ - Just hours after AstraZeneca announced its shot's 79% effectiveness against the virus, the NIAID's Data and Safety Monitoring Board expressed concern that AstraZeneca had included *"outdated information."* NIAID Director Dr. Anthony Fauci oversees the DSMB that assesses trial results and ratifies the board's decisions but is not involved directly in its assessments. He said that the DSMB felt the data released *"might, in fact, be misleading a bit, and wanted them to straighten it out."* The company agreed to set things right soon.

TMR's Take - Americans should be thankful for the independent oversight of the pharmaceutical industry provided by the FDA. AstraZeneca's faulty claim that its vaccine was 79% effective was unnecessary, adding to vaccine hesitancy. Later data confirmed 76% effectiveness. Pfizer has placed enormous resources behind development of a long-lasting, injectable alternative to opioids for pain relief, but the risks unfortunately outweigh the potential benefits. The search for a safe, effective, and non-addictive opioid alternative remains as elusive as the holy grail.

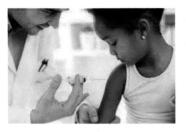

Pfizer to seek authorization for Covid-19 vaccine for children ages 2 to 11 in September, by Naomi Thomas, CNN, 5/4/21

TMR Topline™ - Pfizer expects to file for full FDA approval for its Covid-19 vaccine for people ages 16 to 85 this month and will seek emergency use authorization for its vaccine for children ages 2 to 11 in September. During an earnings call, CEO Albert Bourla also said that Phase 2 safety data from Pfizer's ongoing study in pregnant women is expected by late July or early August.

Full approval will allow Pfizer to market and directly distribute its vaccines. Bourla also stated that Pfizer has submitted information to the FDA that may allow its vaccine to be stored at standard refrigerator temperatures rather than the ultra-cold temperatures required at present.

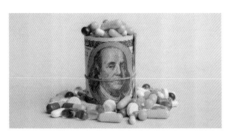

Pfizer posts crazy good quarter with major assist from COVID vaccines, by Tina Reed, Axios, 5/5/21

TMR Topline™ - Pfizer posted about $4.9 billion in 1Q21 profits on revenue of $14.6 billion, up about 45% from $3.4 billion in 1Q20 on revenue of $10.1 billion. It included $3.5 billion in revenue from Pfizer's Covid-19 vaccine that was developed with BioNTech. Pfizer expects sales of its vaccine to total $26 billion for the year, up from an earlier projection of $15 billion. In comparison, Lipitor, one of Pfizer's all-time blockbusters produced annual revenues of $13 billion at its peak.

TMR's Take - Evidence that the Pfizer and Moderna vaccines are safe and effective in children and adolescents is encouraging and should result in millions more Americans being vaccinated. Pfizer stockholders must be ecstatic at its 1Q21 results, a 33.6% profit margin, only a small portion of which goes to federal income taxes. According to the Tax Foundation, Pfizer's federal income tax rate was 6.4% in 2020 compared with 14.6% for the average American taxpayer.

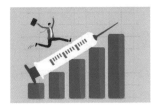

Drugmakers' Spending on Stock, Dividends and Executive Pay Exceeds Research, Democrats Say, by Michael McAuliff, Kaiser Health News, 7/9/21

TMR Topline™ - The report by the House Oversight and Reform Committee found that 14 major drug companies plowed more of their billions in earnings back into their own stocks, dividends and executive compensation ($576 billion) than into R&D ($522 billion) from 2016-2020. Committee Chair Carolyn Maloney (D-N.Y.) stated *"Drug companies are actively and intentionally targeting the United States for price increases, often while cutting prices in the rest of the world."* Moreover, some of that R&D money is spent researching ways to suppress competition, such as by filing hundreds of new, minor patents on older drugs that make it harder to produce generics. H.R. 3, Lower Drug Costs Now Act, would allow Medicare to negotiate drug prices, let Americans with private insurance pay those same rates and limit U.S. prices to an average price other countries pay. Some moderate Democrats raised concerns that it might cut drugmakers' ability to innovate.

According to the report, Novo Nordisk spent twice as much on executive pay and stock buybacks as on R&D over the five years. Amgen spent five times as much on buybacks as on research. An internal presentation from Celgene, which makes the $16,744-a-month cancer drug Revlimid, admitted that it targeted the U.S. for its price hikes because of the country's *"highly favorable environment with free-market pricing."* Internal documents from AbbVie show *"research and development"* being aimed at suppressing cheaper competition, in this case by seeking new minor patent enhancements on the rheumatoid arthritis drug Humira, which costs $77,000 a year. *"An internal presentation on emphasized that one objective of the 'enhancement' strategy was to 'raise barriers to competitor ability to replicate.'"*

Reaction from the industry's lobbying arm, PhRMA, was predictable: *"While we can't speak to specific examples cited in the report, this partisan exercise is clearly designed to garner support for an extreme bill that will erode Medicare protections and access to treatments for seniors."* PhRMA blamed the problem on high deductibles charged by insurers and with profits taken by middlemen such as pharmacy benefit managers.

TMR's Take - On average, prescription drug prices are 2.56 times higher in the U.S. than in 32 other OECD countries. And claiming investments aimed at suppressing cheaper competition as R&D spending is not innovation – quite the opposite. It's an oligopolistic attempt to block competition! The Committee should add those R&D expenses to the more than $100 billion that the industry spent on advertising over the five years to paint a clearer picture of PhRMA's priorities.

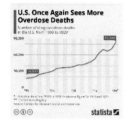

'It's Huge, It's Historic, It's Unheard-of': Drug Overdose Deaths Spike, by Josh Katz and Margot Sanger-Katz, New York Times, 7/14/21

TMR Topline™ - As the Covid pandemic raged, drug abuse deaths rose 30% to more than 93,000 in 2020, disproportionately among the young. Deaths rose in every state but New Hampshire and South Dakota, with the greatest increases in the South and West. A Times analysis estimates that the drug deaths represent 3.5 million years of life compared to 5.5 million for the 375,000 Covid deaths. The pandemic's disruption to outreach and treatment facilities and increased social isolation contributed to the increase as did fentanyls becoming entrenched in the nation's drug supply. Fentanyls are easier to manufacture and ship than traditional heroin with higher potency. The pandemic brought some policy changes that may have saved lives such as allowing people enrolled in methadone treatment to take doses home with them, instead of having to visit a clinic each day. Regulators also made it easier for people to seek medical care through telemedicine.

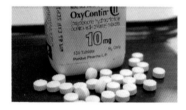

States Announce $26 Billion Settlement to Resolve Opioid Lawsuits, by Sarah Randazzo, Wall Street Journal, 7/21/21

TMR Topline™ - The nation's three largest drug distributors— McKesson Corp. , AmerisourceBergen Corp. , and Cardinal Health Inc. - and drugmaker Johnson & Johnson - have been negotiating the $26 billion deal to resolve thousands of opioid-crisis lawsuits for two years. Under the terms of the settlement, states must spend the funds on social services to address the harms of opioid addiction, like treatment programs, education on disposing pills and needles, and funding for first responders. Over an 18-year period, McKesson will pay up to $7.9 billion, while AmerisourceBergen and Cardinal each agreed to provide up to $6.4 billion. J&J will pay over nine years, with up to $3.7 billion paid during the first three years. The agreement needs support from at least 48 states, 98% of litigating local governments and 97% of the jurisdictions that have yet to sue.

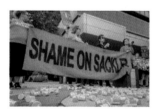

Justice Department Blasts Purdue Pharma's Bankruptcy Plan, by Brian Mann, NPR, 7/19/21

TMR Topline™ - The DoJ is condemning a proposed bankruptcy settlement for Oxycontin maker Purdue Pharma, describing the plan as fatally flawed. Separately, the office of the U.S. Attorney for the SDNY said the plan violated the *"constitutional right to due process"* for those with potential opioid claims. The company's aggressive marketing of Oxycontin that began in the late 1990s is widely seen as a trigger of the nation's deadly opioid epidemic, which has killed more than a half-million Americans. The plan would allow the Sackler family *"third party releases,"* sheltering them from future opioid lawsuits. In return, would contribute roughly $4.3 billion from their private fortunes to help compensate people and communities harmed by Oxycontin.

TMR's Take - The Sackler family earned over $10 billion from Oxycontin and would be relieved of civil and criminal liability if Purdue Pharma's bankruptcy plan is approved. Families of victims are appropriately concerned.

FDA chief Janet Woodcock acknowledges agency may have misstepped in process leading up to Alzheimer's drug approval, by Rachel Cohrs, STAT, 7/14/21

TMR Topline™ - Acting FDA Commissioner Janet Woodcock acknowledged her agency may have misstepped in its handling of its polarizing approval of a new Alzheimer's drug. While defending the therapy and the decision, she said *"it's possible that the process could have been handled in a way that would have decreased the amount of controversy involved."* The agency already has had to narrow the patient population for whom the drug is approved; Woodcock also called for an independent watchdog to investigate the actions that led to the drug's approval. The FDA's approval of Aduhelm has been mired in controversy after controversy since its approval last month amid concerns about a May 2019 off-the-record meeting between an FDA regulator Woodcock supervised and Biogen, the drug's developer.

Will Medicare Pay For The New Alzheimer's Drug?, by Howard Gleckman, Forbes, 7/13/21

TMR Topline™ - Given the FDA approval of Aduhelm, Medicare now must make a National Coverage Determination (NCD) on Biogen's $56,000 a year drug. An independent analysis suggests $3,000-$8,400 would be a reasonable price range. Medicare must determine whether the drug is *"reasonable and necessary for the diagnosis or treatment of illness or injury."* Even if only 1 million of the 6 million Americans with Alzheimer's are prescribed the drug, Medicare costs could exceed $50 billion annually. CMS says it will base its decision on *"an assessment of the clinical evidence such as published clinical studies, professional society guidelines, and public comments."*

TMR's Take - Medicare is not allowed to negotiate drug prices, so Biogen executives and investors will benefit greatly from a positive NCD, even with the narrower approval. Spending at that rate for a drug with unproven effectiveness ultimately could bankrupt Medicare, leaving American taxpayers holding the bag. In a recent issue of *Gooznews*, Modern Healthcare's Editor Emeritus Merrill Goozner argues that Aduhelm is an opportunity for the Patient-Centered Outcomes Research Institute (PCORI) to conduct comparative effectiveness research. Created by the ACA, PCORI conducts studies that measure the *"potential burdens and economic impacts"* of health care services and *"the full range of clinical and patient-centered outcomes."* One arm of the trial would get the unproven drug. Another arm *"would receive home care coupled with non-drug interventions like physical and cognitive exercise. And a third arm would get both."* **TMR** agrees. Such a trial would measure the impact each approach has on cognitive decline as well as how either affects the financial and emotional patients' families well-being. The third arm would determine if the benefits of the two approaches are additive.

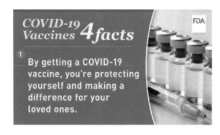

The F.D.A. could grant full approval to Pfizer's vaccine by early September, by Sharon LaFraniere and Noah Weiland, New York Times, 8/4/21

TMR Topline™ - The FDA has accelerated its timetable to fully approve the Pfizer-BioNTech coronavirus vaccine, aiming to complete the process by Labor Day. The agency said its leaders recognized that approval might increase public confidence and had *"taken an all-hands-on-deck approach"* to the work. Recent KFF polls have found that 30% of unvaccinated people said that they would be more likely to take a fully approved vaccine.

TMR's Take - Moderna also has applied for full FDA approval. With full FDA approval, employer vaccine mandates will be on firm legal ground and remove a key reason millions of Americans are delaying vaccination.

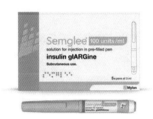

FDA approves use of biosimilar insulin as automatic substitute for costly brand-name, by Aimee Pichee, CBS/AP, 7/29/21

TMR Topline™ - The FDA has given its approval to Semglee, the first biosimilar cleared as a substitute for Lantus, a widely used fast-acting insulin. The FDA agreed that Viatris Inc.'s Semglee was interchangeable with brand name Lantus. Unlike generic drugs, biosimilar drugs are *"highly similar"* duplications. Semglee injector pens cost about $150-190 without insurance for a typical month's supply, compared to $340-520 for the same supply of Lantus. Acting FDA Director Janet Woodcock said: *"This is a momentous day for people who rely daily on insulin for treatment of diabetes, as biosimilar and interchangeable biosimilar products have the potential to greatly reduce health care costs."* **TMR** agrees.

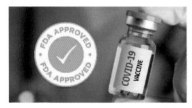

FDA grants full approval to Covid-19 vaccine developed by Pfizer, BioNTech , by Helen Branswell and Andrew Joseph, STAT, 8/23/1

TMR Topline™ - The FDA has granted full approval to the Pfizer/BioNTech Covid-19 vaccine for use in people ages 16 and up. The application was based on a study of 44,000 people, half of whom were given two doses of the Pfizer vaccine. The other half received saline. Based on the six months of follow-up, the vaccine's efficacy in preventing a symptomatic Covid infection was 91.1%. Pfizer's vaccine is sold under the brand name Comirnaty, and 1.2 billion doses have been manufactured so far. Many vaccine-hesitant individuals had cited the EUA as the reason for their reluctance. Full FDA approval removes that excuse and provides firmer ground for public and private organizations to require vaccination.

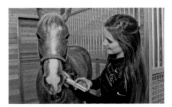

FDA: Stop Using Ivermectin Veterinary Drug to Treat COVID, by Robert Preidt and Robin Foster, WebMD, 8/23/21 (HealthDay News)

TMR Topline™ - After receiving multiple reports of people who have been hospitalized after *"self-medicating with ivermectin intended for horses,"* the FDA has issued a warning that taking a drug meant for horses and cattle to prevent or treat Covid-19 is dangerous and could be fatal. Ivermectin is generally used to treat or prevent parasites in animals. The FDA tweeted *"You are not a horse. You are not a cow. Seriously, y'all. Stop it."* No form of ivermectin has been approved to treat or prevent Covid-19. The Ivermectin tablets and topical formulations for humans have *"very specific doses"* that are significantly smaller than the doses meant for animals.

TMR's Take - The carrot didn't work, but the stick might. The rapid response by public and private organizations to impose vaccine mandates based on the FDA approval may finally move America closer to herd immunity. It's unfortunate that the FDA's limited resources also must deal with the misinformation about Covid-19 being propagated on social media. Last year, it was Hydroxychloroquine; this year it's Ivermectin. Will the dissemination of misinformation ever end?

CHAPTER 8

The Rocky Road to Universal Healthcare in the U.S.

GERMANS HAVE HAD UNIVERSAL HEALTHCARE SINCE 1882. THE OTHER NINE HIGH INCOME COUNTRIES THAT the U.S. is compared with do also, as well as the other 26 member nations of the Organization for Economic Co-operation and Development (OECD). With the most expensive healthcare in the developed world and mediocre outcomes, why is the U.S. such a laggard? Dr. Ashish Jha, the Dean of the Brown University School of Public Health has said, *"The U.S. just isn't much different from other developed countries in how much health care we use. It is very different in how much we pay for it."*

Roughly 30 million Americans are uninsured and another 40 million are underinsured. How did the U.S. reach this abominable state? It wasn't for lack of trying, beginning in 1912 when Theodore Roosevelt ran for President on the Progressive Party ticket. Roosevelt was a fan of the German plan, but his candidacy split the Republican Party and Woodrow Wilson – who had no interest in the issue – was elected President.

The issue remained dormant until Franklin Delano Roosevelt, a distant cousin, was elected President as a Democrat. In completing his cabinet, he offered the post of Secretary of Labor to Frances Perkins, who had worked with him when he was the Governor of New York. She became the first female cabinet member in the United States. She accepted her appointment on the condition that the President back her goals which were to create unemployment insurance; health insurance; old-age insurance, a 40-hour work week; a minimum wage; and abolition of child labor. She later recalled: *"I remember he looked so startled, and he said, 'Well, do you think it can be done?'"* She promised to find out.

FDR's legislative accomplishments were transformative in lifting the economy from the depths of the Great Depression, but universal healthcare fell by the wayside. Faced with strong opposition from the American Medical Association, Roosevelt had to drop healthcare in order to secure passage of the Social Security Act in 1935. World War II brought with it wage and price controls. Some industries vital to the war effort were unable to recruit employees due to their remote location (e.g., Kaiser Steel's new plant in Fontana California, 90 miles east of Los

Angeles). In 1942, the War Labor Board decided to allow employers to offer fringe benefits to help attract and retain workers. That changed everything.

Employers began offering health insurance coverage as nontaxable compensation for their workers. In 1954, the Internal Revenue Service ruled that the cost of health insurance was not taxable to the employee. In effect, the road to a government operated single payer system like the U.K's National Health Service was now blocked.

Following FDR's death in 1945 and his election to a full term in 1948, President Harry Truman tried to include health care as a part of his Fair Deal Plan. Once again, strong opposition to "socialized medicine" from the American Medical Association defeated the proposal. When he left office in 1952, Truman said that his biggest disappointment was his inability to establish a national health program during his years in the White House.

The issue remained dormant for another 13 years until Lyndon Baines Johnson became President after President Kennedy was assassinated. In 1965, both Medicare and Medicaid were enacted as part of his "Great Society" program. Today, these programs serve more than 143 million Americans.

William Jefferson Clinton was elected President in 1992 after campaigning heavily on healthcare reform. After taking office, he appointed First Lady Hillary Clinton to head up a multifaceted task force to devise a plan for universal healthcare. The task force of over 500 people on 34 committees including academics; executives from the insurance, hospital and pharmaceutical industries; physicians; representatives of business and assorted policy makers – met in secret for 9 months and produced a complex proposal for "managed competition" to provide universal healthcare for all Americans. Bogged down by its complexity and vigorously opposed by the insurance industry's highly effective series of "Harry & Louise" TV ads, HR 1200, the Health Security Act was dead on arrival when it reached Congress.

Later, in Clinton's second term, the Balanced Budget Act of 1997 created the Children's Health Insurance Program (CHIP). CHIP is a state-federal partnership that provides health insurance to low-income children; 9.6 million children are currently enrolled. However, real healthcare reform would have to wait another generation until Barack Obama took office in 2009.

Like Clinton, President Obama was committed to improving access to healthcare in America. At the time of his inauguration, 50 million Americans were uninsured. He tried for months to gain bipartisan support for improving access to health insurance, but Republicans, especially Iowa's Senator Chuck Grassley, remained intransigent. The Patient Protection and Affordable Care Act was enacted in 2010 without a single Republican vote. To secure passage, the proposal for a public option had to be dropped from the bill. Today more than 20 million Americans have health insurance coverage through this program despite more than 60 attempts to "Repeal and Replace Obamacare" during the last ten years.

In his first 100 days in office, President Joe Biden worked to secure passage of the American Rescue Plan Act (ARPA) that provides a framework to lead the country out of the pandemic induced recession. ARPA has been hailed as the largest improvement in healthcare since the passage of the ACA. It includes subsidies to reduce the cost of insurance for those who are eligible based on income levels, and it provides the opportunity to expand Medicaid coverage in the 12 states that have not yet done so. This aspect of the ARPA is set to expire in two years. The Commonwealth Fund projects that if these improvements to the ACA are made permanent by future legislation, it would reduce the number of uninsured by 7 million and would increase the federal budget by an additional $442 billion over the next ten years. If the projection is accurate, there still would be 14 million uninsured Americans.

Achieving universal healthcare for all Americans is a divisive issue; in general, Democrats believe that access to affordable, quality healthcare is a fundamental human right, not a privilege for those who can afford it. Republicans grouse about the costs of providing government-supported healthcare as socialism. The first book in this series, "Healing American Healthcare, A Plan to Provide Quality Care For All While Saving $1 Trillion A Year," set forth the Eichhorn Hutchinson Allcare Plan that provides a framework for an affordable universal healthcare plan for America. In summary it includes the following:

- A lower cost public option based on Medicare that would compete with private insurance.
- All employers would be required to provide health insurance for their employees. They could use private insurance, the public option or they could be self-insured.
- Individuals could also purchase the public option.
- Employed Medicaid beneficiaries would be covered by their employers; thus, Medicaid would no longer provide subsidies under Obamacare for self-insured low-income employees because they would be covered by employment supplied insurance.
- Establish a national drug negotiating plan as other nations have done and allow Medicare Part D to begin negotiating drug prices.
- It would establish a standard reimbursement rate for provider reimbursement above the Medicare schedule and would reduce the administrative complications and the cost of billing for medical and prescription services.
- It would require electronic healthcare record interoperability and replace preauthorization requirements of public and private insurance plans with post payment review to ferret out fraud.

This plan could reduce Federal budget Medicaid expenses by more than $300 billion annually. It has been estimated that allowing Medicare to negotiate drug prices could also save an additional $80 billion per year. It provides an opportunity for strategic compromise between Democrats and Republicans. It promotes choice and competition while providing a major budget reduction that should appeal to most Republicans while providing universal access to affordable, quality healthcare that Democrats support. A more detailed review of the plan is provided in Appendix A.

The 12 articles summarized in this chapter cover the following topics, including:

- Pandemic inspired universal healthcare approaches and issues.
- Democratic efforts and plans to improve healthcare.
- U.S. healthcare performance compared with other high-income nations.

Universal Healthcare Three Minute Reads

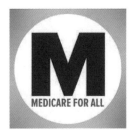

Improving the prognosis of health care in the USA, by Alison P Galvani, Alyssa S Parpia, Eric M Foster, Burton H Singer, Meagan C Fitzpatrick, The Yale School of Public Health. The Lancet 2/15/20

TMR Topline™ - The study's authors estimate that Medicare-for-All could save $450 billion annually with $188 billion coming from reduced payments to hospitals and physicians. The reduced income for physicians would be offset by eliminating bad debt and reducing bureaucracy since all would be covered, including 40 million Americans who are currently uninsured or underinsured.

TMR's Take - The Yale study has material shortcomings. For one, it fails to estimate the financial impact on physician practices of a.) the tradeoffs of reducing bad debt and bureaucracy b.) eliminating private insurance and Medicaid and c.) caring for 40 million more patients seeking medical care. Flawed as it may be the study was quoted repeatedly by Senator Sanders to justify his Medicare-for-All proposal in speeches and debates during the Presidential primary season.

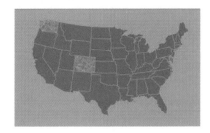

COVID-19 pandemic weakens push for public option, by Rich Daly, HFMA senior writer and editor, 6/16/20

TMR Topline™ - Colorado and Washington state have either halted or slowed their launch of public option plans. The decisions to throttle back the plans were spurred by providers' financial challenges amid the pandemic. Colorado's plan required hospital participation and set minimum provider payment rates at 155% of Medicare rates. Washington's Cascade Care set most provider rates at 160% of Medicare rates.

TMR's Take - The pandemic-induced delay to implement a public option is unfortunate. The Eichhorn-Hutchinson universal healthcare plan provides choice along with a public option, and reduces administrative waste, drug costs and medically related bankruptcies. HFMA

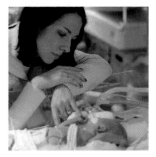

Association of Air Pollution and Heat Exposure With Preterm Birth, Low Birth Weight, and Stillbirth in the US: A Systematic Review, by Bruce Bekkar, MD; Susan Pacheco, MD; Rupa Basu, PhD; Nathaniel DeNicola, MD, MSHP, JAMA Open Net, 6/18/20

TMR Topline™ - The authors reviewed 57 studies from 2007 through 2019 that included more than 32 million U.S. births and found that pregnant women exposed to air pollution and/or high temperatures are more likely to give birth to babies who are premature, underweight, or stillborn. Their review strongly suggests that the toll on babies' health will grow as climate change worsens. Other key findings include:

- The risks are higher for minority women: Black women are 2.4 times more likely to have low birth weight babies than white women.

- Higher temperatures were linked to an increased risk of premature birth and lower birth weight.

- One study found that from May to September, temperature increases the week before delivery increased the possibility of a stillbirth.

- Most of the studies concluded that exposure to air pollution was also associated with preterm births, low birth weights and stillbirth.

- Living closer to power plants was also reported as a high risk for preterm births.

- Asthmatic mothers exposed to high levels of air pollution were 52% more likely to give birth prematurely.

- The risks are compounded in minority communities that have less access to medical care.

- Minority patients tend not to receive the same level of treatment than women who live in more affluent communities.

TMR's Take Premature birth and low birthweight can have lasting effects on brain development and vulnerability to disease. The authors concluded that "*This really does set the stage for an entire generation.*" To address this growing problem, the U.S. must reinstate efforts to control air pollution, revitalize plans to address global warming and establish fairness in healthcare through the development of a Universal Healthcare program like the Eichhorn-Hutchinson Allcare plan that provides choice along with a public option and reduces administrative waste, drug costs and medically related bankruptcies. None of these important efforts will be easy: all demand our attention.

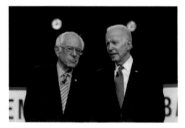

Biden-Sanders task force health platform pushes for public option, a free COVID-19 vaccine, by Paige Minemyer, Fierce Healthcare, 7/9/2020

TMR Topline™ - The platform released by presumptive Democratic presidential nominee places a high priority on implementing a public option, including a plan with no deductible. Building on the ACA, Medicare, Medicaid and the VA system, the healthcare task force members wrote "*Private insurers need real competition to ensure they have incentive to provide affordable, quality coverage to every American.*" Co-chaired by Rep. Pramila Jayapal, D-Washington, and former Surgeon General Vivek Murthy, M.D., the task force's principal recommendations also include:

- Make free Covid-19 testing more widely available and, when available, vaccines for the virus to come at no cost to the patient.

- Recruit 100,000 contact tracers and set up a system for public health agencies to track the virus.

- Set a cap to ensure that patients spend no more than 8.5% of their income on premiums and lift the cap on subsidies for ACA plans.

- Allow Medicare to negotiate directly with drug manufacturers on pricing, and cap out-of-pocket drug costs for seniors.

- Lower the age for Medicare enrollment to 60.

TMR's Take - In speeches and articles last year, your Editor forecast that "M4A is DOA" and the task force co-chaired by one of its most ardent advocates saw the light. Their approach has much in common with the Eichhorn-Hutchinson universal healthcare plan that provides choice along with a public option, and reduces administrative waste, drug costs and medically related bankruptcies. Other than continued efforts to repeal the ACA, Republicans have yet to release their healthcare plan.

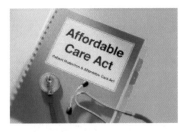

Overturning the ACA Would Increase Uninsurance among People of All Ages, Races and Ethnicities, by Linda J. Blumberg, The Urban Institute, 10/20/20

TMR Topline™ - The Supreme Court will begin to hear arguments 11/10 on the constitutionality of the Accountable Care Act (ACA) in the case of California v. Texas. A group of Republican state attorneys general argue that passage of a 2017 tax law that eliminated the ACA's individual mandate penalties renders the entire ACA unconstitutional. The Trump administration supports their position. This case is being opposed by a group led by the California attorney general. The Urban Institute analyzed the potential impact if the Supreme Court overturns the ACA and found the following:

- 21.1 million Americans would be uninsured in 2022.

- 9.3 million people would lose their income related health insurance subsidies in 2022.

- Medicaid and CHIP coverage would decline by 15.5 million people in 2022.

- Federal government spending on health care would decrease by $152 billion per year.

- Healthcare coverage will fall for people of all races and ethnicities in every state.

The ACA's protection for preexisting conditions and coverage age limits for adult children also would be eliminated. Hospitals, physicians, and pharmaceutical companies will experience large decreases in revenue. The positive aspects of increased coverage achieved under the ACA will be reversed. It is hard to quantify the total impact of the law being judged unconstitutional because almost all insurers, providers, and households would be affected by the elimination of the ACA's many provisions.

TMR's Take - If the ACA is overturned by the Supreme Court in California v. Texas, policymakers and the next Congress will have to find an acceptable way to replace this law to prevent an economic and healthcare crisis in 2022.

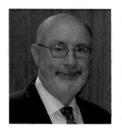

Strategic Compromise – The Pathway to Universal Healthcare,
The Healing American Healthcare Coalition Blog by Ed Eichhorn 1/3/21

TMR Topline™ - Healthcare in America should be a right and not just a privilege for those who can afford it. In the current political environment, universal healthcare appears to be unattainable, however we can achieve what every other democracy in the world has achieved by building a strategic compromise.

Over the last 110 years at least ten presidents have been expressed interest in expanding healthcare coverage. However only Presidents Johnson and Obama were successful in introducing major legislation that expanded health insurance coverage for large segments of the population. President Johnson succeeded in passing Medicare and Medicaid legislation in 1965 and President Obama was successful in passing the Affordable Care Act in 2009. Today these programs provide health insurance coverage for almost 140 million Americans.

What would a strategic compromise look like today? The progressive Democrats want universal healthcare, Historically Republicans prefer programs that reduce the deficit. If the United States would adapt the German System, all employers would have to provide health insurance for their employees. Prior to the pandemic, 16% of Medicaid beneficiaries were employed. If their employers provided them with health insurance, the federal expense for Medicaid would be reduced by more than $200 billion per year.

This is the strategic compromise. The Democrats get universal healthcare for America, and the Republicans get reduced federal and state expenses for Medicaid. More importantly we would significantly improve healthcare outcomes for all Americans by making healthcare a right and not just a privilege.

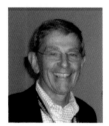

America First? On Health, America's Worst!, The Healing American
Healthcare Coalition Blog by John Dalton, FHFMA, 2/28/21

TMR Topline™ - Last week's CPAC meeting touted former President Trump's *"America First"* policy. When it comes to America's health, that thought could hardly be further from the truth. Updated Commonwealth Fund data shows America as the biggest spender with the worst outcomes among 11 high income OECD members:

- The U.S. spent 17.0% of GDP on healthcare; OECD average 8.8%; range 9.3-12.1%.
- The U.S. spent $10,637 per capita; OECD average $4,224, range $4,205-7,732.
- Average life expectancy 78.7 years U.S.; OECD average 80.7, highest, Switzerland 83.1.
- The U.S. also was highest for suicide rate/100,000 vs. OECD average (14.5 vs. 11.2), adults with multiple chronic conditions (29.0% vs. 17.7%) and obesity (40% vs. 24%).
- The U.S. Covid-19 fatality rate of 154.8/100,000 is 41.6% above the OECD average of 109.3/100,000 at 2/28/21.

Last month, Lancet released the report of its Commission on Public Policy and Health in the Trump Era, concluding: *"The suffering and dislocation inflicted by Covid-19 has exposed the frailty of the US social and medical order, and the interconnectedness of society. A new politics is needed, whose appeal rests on a vision of shared prosperity and a kind society. Healthcare workers have much to contribute in formulating and advancing that vision, and our patients, communities, and planet have much to gain from it.*" The Eichhorn-Hutchinson Allcare plan depicts one such vision, providing a practical path to universal healthcare for all Americans. Like Bidencare, it builds on the strengths of the Affordable Care Act without the economic disruptions of Medicare-For-All. Allcare relies on competition and choice, and includes a public option based on Medicare.

TMR's Take - It's time for all Americans to unite behind moving America's healthcare system from worst to first!

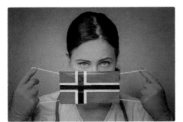

Crisis Showcases Corner of Europe Derided by Trump Advisers, by Niclas Rolander and Ott Umelas, Bloomberg Business Week, 1/11/21

TMR Topline™ - In its 2018 report "*The Opportunity Costs of Socialism,*" President Trump's advisers trashed the Nordic economic model saying it reduced living standards. One year into the worst global pandemic in more than a century, the World Economic Forum credits the region's societal model as "*the most promising*" in charting a sustainable path out of the crisis.

Bloomberg Economics Johanna Jeansson points out that these small export-oriented nations had certain advantages including "*deep public coffers, a tight social security net, and a larger reliance on sectors that have been able to work from home and sell online.*" With low levels of debt as a percent of GDP (Denmark and Sweden – 40%; Finland – 70%; EU average – 90%), the countries have more leeway to spend their way out of the coronavirus recession. HSBC Economist James Pomeroy said: "*If you have a very digitally savvy population, that sets you up very well going forward in terms of productivity.*"

TMR's Take - TMR's 1/7/21 podcast, "*Covid-19 2020 – which countries protected their residents best?*" reviews results for the 37 OECD member nations and others, highlights former CDC Director Dr. Tom Frieden's selections for best in various categories and adds **TMR's** choice for best in Europe: **Norway**, with a year-end fatality rate of 8.12/100,000, fifth in the OECD.

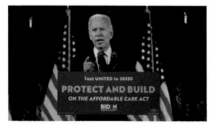

Healthcare industry gearing up to try to find common ground with Biden, by Lola Butcher, Modern Healthcare, 3/8/21

TMR Topline™ - The healthcare industry agrees with the Biden administration: the current top priority must be the Covid-19 pandemic along with increasing insurance coverage. Biden's primary strategy to decrease the percentage of uninsured is to revitalize the ACA. Last month, lobbies representing providers, payers, and employers, formed the Affordable Coverage Coalition (ACC) whose goal is to achieve universal health coverage through several steps. These include enhancing the ACA premium subsidies and providing incentives for more states to expand Medicaid. The ACC does not agree with two of the President's campaign promises: creating a public option that would allow people to buy into Medicare and reducing the Medicare eligibility age to 60.

A 2019 AHA and FAH study suggested that a government-run, Medicare-like option would lead to nearly $800 million in provider payment cuts over 10 years while utilization was growing. The Medicare Trust Fund is projected to have insufficient funds to cover its obligations beginning in 2024. Commonwealth Fund CEO Dr. David Blumenthal said: *""If the Congress wants to give more people the coverage that Medicare offers, there are ways to fund it—it's just a matter of finding the political will to do so,"*

Noting that telehealth has made healthcare more accessible and affordable, especially in rural communities, AHA's Ashley Thompson, Senior Vice President for Policy said: *"We are going to need help from Congress to remove some of the key barriers in order to make telehealth continue being used as it has during the public health emergency."* There is bi-partisan support on this issue as well as on drug pricing. A PhRMA representative stated that any *"government price setting"* is a bright line that the drug industry is unwilling to cross. The industry's success in vaccine development to combat the Covid-19 pandemic may give it the political power it needs to fight drug pricing controls.

The pandemic has severely strained America's healthcare workforce. The December Covid-19 relief bill authorized Medicare to fund 1,000 additional physician residency slots. The Association of American Medical Colleges predicts a shortage of up to 139,000 physicians by 2033 and sees this as an opportunity to begin to address the projected shortage. Biden's Covid-relief plan provides funding for 100,000 public health workers.

TMR's Take - A recent Populace study found that across race, gender, income, education, generation, and 2020 presidential vote, there is agreement on America's long-term national priorities. Chief among them: high quality healthcare as a necessity, not a privilege; an overwhelming commitment to individual rights; and upholding equal treatment for all, but not necessarily equal outcomes. President Biden created a Covid-19 Health Equity Task Force that is recommending equitable allocation of Covid-related resources and funds. The task force must also develop a long-term plan to improve data collection for communities of color and other underserved populations.

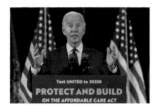

Democrats in both chambers launch public option effort, by Mary Ellen McIntire, ROLL CALL, 5/26/21

TMR Topline™ - Senate Health, Education, Labor and Pensions Chair Patty Murray, D-Wash. and House Energy and Commerce Chair Frank Pallone, Jr., D-N.J., recently issued a request for information asking for input on a public option, which would establish a government-run health plan to compete with private insurers. *"Our goal in establishing a federally administered public option is to work towards achieving universal coverage, while making health care simpler and more affordable for patients and families,"* they wrote. Democrats in both chambers have proposed different bills that would establish a public option, but Murray and Pallone indicated they would develop a new proposal. They will have a difficult time passing legislation to enact a public option because Democrats have a very slim majority in Congress. Although the Senate Democrats could use the reconciliation process to pass public option legislation without Republican support, it would require no defections among Senate Democrats.

Senators Tim Kaine, D-Va., and Michael Bennett, D-Colo. said, *"We are glad to see a public option gaining momentum in the Senate. Over the last five years, we have worked to draft the Medicare-X Choice Act, which we believe is the best public option proposal available. We look forward to working with the Biden Administration and our Senate leadership and colleagues in moving a public option forward to bring us one step closer to achieving universal health care in this country."*

TMR Take – TMR agrees that the passage of a public option is the important next step towards universal coverage in America since it will foster competition for subscribers. The insurance lobby is funding the Partnership for America's Health Care Future to fight public option proposals in Colorado and Connecticut. Why? They don't want a new competitor that might disrupt their profitable insurance market.

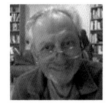

The All-Payer Pricing Alternative, by Merrill Goozner, Gooznews, 6/8/21

TMR Topline™ - In a lengthy article, Modern Healthcare's Editor Emeritus discusses some of the alternate routes to reaching a public option being pursued by several states as well as their critical flaws. For example, Washington's Cascade Care set benefit standards and payment rates (at 160% of Medicare) for an additional plan that private insurers must sell and administer if they want to participate on the exchange. It was the low-cost option in just 8 of the state's 39 counties. Instead, Goozner suggests all-payer pricing and explores the Maryland system – all-payer pricing combined with global budgeting – that has operated under a federal waiver since 1974. Different hospitals are allowed to charge different rates based on their historic baselines but cannot charge different patients different rates based on the insurance card they carry. RTI International's recent analysis looked at FYs 2011 to 2018: *"Depending on the year and basis for comparison, Medicare payment rates for inpatient rates were 33 to 44 percent higher under Maryland's all-payer rate-setting system."* Commercial insurance rates were 11-15% lower than in a matched comparison group. To eliminate incentives for unnecessary utilization, global budgeting was added in 2014. Those budgets are increased each year based on inflation, changes in population and other factors.

Maryland's all-payer pricing system increased federal spending but allowed commercial insurers to lower premiums by double digit rates. When coupled with a global budgeting, all-payer pricing slowed the growth of health care spending. Maryland's benchmark premium rates have fallen by 29% for private plans sold on Maryland's Obamacare exchange from 2018-21, 23% below the national average. Goozner cites the following advantages of all-payer/global budgeting:

- Sharply reduces administrative waste by eliminating the multiple pricing schedules and billing systems inside hospitals and insurance companies;
- Lowers premiums for employer group plans and for individual plans sold on the exchanges; and
- Incentivizes hospitals to compete on efficiency, quality, service, safety and outcomes.

Dr. John Chessare, CEO of Greater Baltimore Medical Center said: *"Those of us who have drank the Kool-Aid are deploying the resources into patient-centered medical homes, behavioral health, sexual assault forensic examination programs. We're spending money in the outpatient area to drive better value."*

TMR Take – Creative well-studied approaches to reduce hospital and private insurance costs that promote competition on quality, efficiency and outcomes need to be part of the future of healthcare in America.

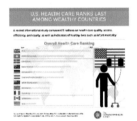

US comes in last in health care rankings of high-income countries, by Tami Luhby, CNN, 8/4/21

TMR Topline™ - The U.S. once again ranked last among 11 high-income countries (Australia, Canada, France, Germany, the Netherlands, New Zealand, Norway, Sweden, Switzerland and the U.K.). The Commonwealth Fund's 7th study since 2004 has consistently ranked the U.S. last overall. Norway, the Netherlands and Australia ranked best. The U.S. ranked last in access to health care, equity and outcomes despite spending 16.8% of GDP on healthcare compared with a range of 9.1-11.7% of GDP by the other 10 countries (2019 data). It is the only one not to have universal health insurance coverage.

TMR's Take - Five years ago, your Editor wrote a three-part series, *"American Healthcare – Worst Value in the Developed World?"* documenting concerns that, despite having the best-equipped hospitals and most thoroughly trained physicians, the U.S. delivers high-cost care of mediocre quality. Sadly, little has changed, and the U.S. has the highest infant and maternal mortality rates among the 11 high-income countries, as well as the highest rate of avoidable deaths and lowest life expectancy at age 60.

CHAPTER 9

Lessons from the Pandemic

THE COVID-19 PANDEMIC PLACED ENORMOUS PRESSURE ON AMERICA'S HEALTHCARE DELIVERY SYSTEM, exposing many weaknesses that need to be addressed before the next outbreak. With five major outbreaks thus far in the 21st century (SARS, MERS, Swine Flu, Ebola and Covid-19), it's not if, but when. All were concerns pre-pandemic. They include:

- America must continue shifting healthcare's emphasis from treating diseases to promoting health.
- Telehealth filled a vital gap during the pandemic; let's make sure that it's here to stay.
- China is not America's friend. Its lack of full cooperation with the World Health Organization's investigation impeded the global response.
- Offshoring the manufacture of critical elements in the supply chain led to critical shortages.
- Burnout among frontline clinicians is endemic. Post-pandemic, who will be left to care for us?
- Consistent leadership commitment to protecting their residents is crucial to containing outbreaks, whether at federal, state or local levels. Letting politics trump public health is unacceptable.
- Longer term, America would do well to emulate the Scandinavians, whose countries controlled Covid-19 better than most and consistently rank among the happiest people in the world in annual surveys.

This final chapter offers some closing thoughts on each of these subjects with the hope that U.S. policy makers will have the courage and commitment to address them.

From curing disease to promoting health

WITH THE BEST-EQUIPPED HOSPITALS and most thoroughly trained physicians, America excels at treating and curing disease. This again was evident in the early stages of the pandemic when fully engaged clinicians were learning on the fly. In America's most densely populated state, New Jersey hospitals worked collaboratively with each other and state officials to develop models and methodologies to guide a data-driven and formulaic approach to sharing and utilizing information to beat back the virus. Learning on the fly, Chief Medical Officers and Chief Nursing Officers held daily teleconferences to share successes and failures, discussing what treatments and protocols worked well and what should be set aside. The collaborative approach worked. In April 2020, a patient hospitalized with Covid-19 had a 26.7% likelihood of death. By February 2021, that likelihood had dropped to 11.4%.

Similarly, the case fatality rate (# of deaths / # of cases x 100) was 8.2% at April 30, 2020. That percentage might be slightly overstated as testing was not widely prevalent then. By year end, it had declined to 2.2% and has continued to decline. At August 30, 2021, it was 1.9%, a 13.6% improvement over 2020's year end.

However, the U.S. has consistently ranked last in the Commonwealth Fund's periodic healthcare rankings for 11 high income countries (Australia, Canada, France, Germany, the Netherlands, New Zealand, Norway, Sweden, Switzerland and the U.K.). Why the paradox? The World Health Organization defines *health* as *"a state of complete physical, mental and **social** well-being."* The other ten countries that consistently outrank the U.S. have more comprehensive social services safety nets that, among other factors, support public health initiatives in their communities.

An article summary in an earlier chapter highlighted the efforts being undertaken by New Jersey's RWJBarnabas Health to address these shortcomings with its "Health Beyond the Hospital" initiative. Its objectives include referring and connecting patients to community-based services in addressing the social determinants of health (SDOH). The goal is to assess patients' risk factors for chronic disease by removing the stigma around questioning housing, safety, and nutrition. After the initial screening, the Health Beyond the Hospital program uses a community referral platform to connect people with services personalized to meet their health and social needs based on age, gender, eligibility, location, primary language, and insurance coverage.

Health systems that succeed in providing better care while improving healthy behaviors in the communities they serve will lower the per capita costs of care and produce better outcomes on the key health indicators. That's the Triple Aim, and America has a long road ahead to achieve it.

Telehealth must be here to stay

AMERICA'S MEDICAL PRACTICES RAPIDLY pivoted to telehealth as a care delivery mechanism at the outset of the pandemic and payers agreed to reimburse visits at office visit rates. It proved to be an effective substitute for in-office visits for a wide range of conditions. For example, from March-July 2020 telehealth consultations successfully diverted millions of dollars of SNF transfers. Instead of calling 911 and shipping an ailing resident off to a hospital emergency room, most of the frail elderly were diagnosed and treated without the disruption of an ambulance ride to the nearest hospital.

Frail elderly patients and those in rural areas for whom travel to a doctor's office is a challenge found that telehealth proved a real blessing. Parents leery of bringing a sick child to a pediatrician's office crowded with other sick children found that an on-line visit was just what the doctor ordered in most instances. Clinicians became very creative finding ways to diagnose from afar.

The Centers for Medicare and Medicaid Services (CMS) estimates that more than 94% of Medicare Advantage plans will offer telehealth benefits next year, up from 58% of plans in 2020.

In the April 2021 Senate confirmation hearing for President Biden's nominee for CMS Administrator, Senator Ron Wyden (D-Ore.), chairman of the Finance Committee, said: *"As a result of the pandemic, we've removed some of the roadblocks for people to actually get to a telehealth provider. We're going to have to make those kinds of changes permanent in addition to working on the critical reimbursement issue."*

Other Committee members echoed Wyden's comments, noting that it is an area of potential bipartisan agreement.

Deployed effectively, telehealth is a cost-effective way to deliver patient-centric care, particularly to frail elderly for whom travel is a challenge and those in rural areas.

China is not America's friend

WHETHER DUE TO EMBARRASSMENT that *"wildlife wet markets"* still existed in China or that the SARS-CoV-2 virus resulted from an accidental lab leak from the Wuhan Institute of Virology, China's government has been less than fully cooperative in working with the World Health Organization (WHO) to determine its origin.

A research study of four Wuhan markets conducted by virologist Xiao Xiao from 5/17-11/19 found that nearly 1/3 of the animals he examined bore trapping and shooting wounds consistent with being caught in the wild, and included masked palm civets, raccoon dogs, bamboo rats, minks and hog badgers.

Such animals are a well-known path for zoonotic disease transmission. A spillover from a wet market in Guangdong caused the 2003 SARS outbreak.

The WHO is setting up a Scientific Advisory Group for the Origins of Novel Pathogens, or SAGO to help establish frameworks for investigating the origins of pathogens early on as cases of disease are reported, as well as determining the origins of SARS-CoV-2.

For the U.S., the adage, *"Keep your friends close and your enemies closer"* may apply.

Critical supplies should be on shored

ORDINARY AMERICANS HAVE LEARNED a lot of new words since the beginning of the pandemic including such esoteric terms as "anosmia," the loss of the sense of smell that was a clear indicator of a potential Covid-19 infection. However, "supply chain" may have been the most important term to enter the vernacular during the pandemic, along with the overworked "pivot" and "unprecedented."

For Americans used to abundance and variety when grocery shopping, the sight of empty shelves was shocking. Toilet paper shortages were one thing, but more critical were the shortages of personal protective equipment (PPE), reagents and other materials crucial to battling the pandemic. Why? In most instances, these items were being manufactured offshore to take advantage of lower labor costs.

While the media showed images of frontline healthcare workers reusing N95 masks and wearing garbage bags due to a shortage of gowns, replacement supplies ordered from overseas often were diverted to higher bidders or retained for use in the country where they were manufactured. Other critical items in short supply included gloves, face shields and ventilators.

Necessity is the mother of invention, and the media was replete with stories about how American companies, many whose business had been adversely affected by the pandemic, pivoted to reconfigure their processes to meet the need. It still took months to develop an adequate supply. There also were far too many stories of "pandemic profiteers" taking advantage of the crisis to bilk providers.

The Lown Institute's 2020 1st place in its annual Shkreli Awards (named for the entrepreneur who raised the price of Daraprim from $13.50 to $750 a pill in 2015) went to Jared Kushner and the federal government's Project Airbridge, to *"airlift PPE from overseas and bring it to the U.S. quickly"* to go to designated pandemic hotspots. Instead, the supplies were given to six private medical supply companies to sell to the highest bidder, setting off a bidding war among the states. No officials from the 10 hardest hit counties said that they received PPE from Project Airbridge.

Preparing to meet the challenges of the next outbreak will require "onshoring" the manufacture of certain critical supply items even if at a higher cost.

Clinician shortages and burnout must be addressed

PRIOR TO THE PANDEMIC, America faced a shortage of 15,000 primary care physicians; federal data shows that 82 million Americans live in primary care *"health professional shortage areas."*

An August 2020 Physicians Foundation survey found that burnout increased from 40% to 58% since the 2018 survey and 38% of physicians want to retire in the next year.

The Bureau of Labor Statistics projects that 176,000 new nurses will be needed annually yet nursing schools don't have enough faculty to expand the nursing work force.

A Health Affairs study found that the average rate of nursing home staff turnover is more than 100% per year. The turnover rate for registered nurses was 140.7% while the rate for licensed practical nurses and certified nursing assistants was 114.1%.

With 10,000 Baby Boomers turning 65 every day, who will be there to care for them?

Committed compassionate leadership is key

ARGUABLY, THE MOST IMPORTANT issue to be addressed has to do with leadership. The onset of the Covid-19 pandemic caught most countries unprepared and leadership responses varied greatly. Scholars will spend the next generation dissecting the nuances of type of governing structure, level of preparedness and other variables in their doctoral dissertations. In the metrics-driven co-authors opinion, the type of governance structure mattered much less than the compassionate commitment of the head of state to protect the country's residents from Covid-19, placing public health above political considerations.

When America needed competent, thoughtful, and decisive elected leadership to guide the planning and actions taken to meet and defeat the challenge, President Trump attempted to downplay the threat in public comments and tweets. On February 27th , he predicted: *"It's going to disappear. One day it's like a miracle, it will disappear."* The next day, at a South Carolina rally, he referred to the coronavirus as the Democrats' *"new hoax."*

While countries throughout the world looked to America's Centers for Disease Control and Prevention (CDC) for leadership and advice, Trump chose to ignore it. In April, President Trump stopped funding of the World Health Organization, accusing it of *"severely mismanaging and covering up the spread of the virus."* At a news conference, later that month he suggested injecting bleach as a potential coronavirus treatment. The FDA quickly refuted this outrageous suggestion.

Placing politics above public health, he left implementation of mitigation measures to the governors of each state. Predictably, the results varied widely. In areas hit hard early, mitigation measures were adopted. America's first confirmed Covid-19 case was in Washington state as well as the first major outbreak in a Kirkland nursing home. Yet, Washington has consistently had fatality rates below the OECD average. When Metro New York joined Milan and Madrid as the global epicenters of the pandemic, the governors of Connecticut, New Jersey and New York collaborated daily to battle the pandemic, learning on the fly.

Other governors chose to ignore HHS Secretary Alex Azar's advice to *"Wash your hands, watch your distance and wear a mask."* Texas Governor Greg Abbot allowed bars and restaurants to reopen two weeks before Memorial Day 2020. It resulted in a large uptick in infections by mid-June. Florida Governor Ron DeSantis kept health clubs open without restrictions because people who go to them are physically active and healthy. Members got sick. Florida's beaches remained open during Spring Break leading to infections at many colleges in other states after the partiers returned to campus. In fall 2020, DeSantis insisted that all schools open with a normal five day a week schedule and threatened to withhold school aid if they did not. This year, he threatened to not pay superintendents who required masks to protect their students. Like DeSantis, Abbot opposes mask mandates.

South Dakota Governor Kristi Noem allowed the annual Sturgis Motorcycle Rally to draw nearly 500,000 to the small South Dakota town from August 7-16, 2020. Rallygoers filled bars, restaurants, concert venues and tattoo parlors with many going unmasked. By mid-September, more than 330 cases and one death were causally linked to the rally and the Dakotas, along with Wyoming, Minnesota and Montana, were leading the nation in new coronavirus infections per capita. Experts agree that the total number of cases will never be known since contact tracing doesn't always capture the source of the infection and asymptomatic spread goes unnoticed. Kaiser Family Foundation epidemiologist Josh Michaud said: *"Holding a half-million-person rally in the midst of a pandemic is emblematic of a nation as a whole that maybe isn't taking [the novel coronavirus] as seriously as we should."*

President Trump did invoke the Defense Production Act to require Ford Motor Company to make ventilators. He did not use it to expand the PPE supply. States and hospital systems ended up bidding against each other to get the supplies that they needed. For many months, disposable supplies had to be reused for extended periods of time.

He erroneously announced that the FDA had approved the anti-malaria drug, hydroxychloroquine, for treating Covid-19. Used for treatment of lupus and arthritis, demand for the drug grew based on the President's recommendation. That led to shortages for those who relied on hydroxychloroquine for treatment of their chronic illnesses. In July, the FDA stipulated that it should not be used outside of a hospital setting to treat Covid patients given its likelihood to cause cardiac arrythmia.

Operation Warp Speed, a public-private partnership to encourage the development of safe, effective vaccines, diagnostics and therapeutics was announced May 5. It was a major success. Pfizer/BioNTech and Moderna (in partnership with the vaccine experts at the NIH) developed mRNA-based vaccines in less than a year. That scientific breakthrough is the 21st century equivalent of the Salk and Sabin vaccines that defeated polio in the 1950s. Johnson & Johnson's single dose adenovirus vaccine from its Janssen Pharmaceuticals subsidiary also proved to be safe and effective.

Unfortunately, plans were not made for the complex logistical challenges of distributing and administering the vaccines. By the time Trump left office, only 16 million doses had been administered. Had President Trump merely listened to his public health experts, hundreds of thousands of American deaths could have been avoided. As of January 31, 2020, the U.S. ranked 32nd of 37 among the OECD's member nations. Had the U.S. merely matched the OECD average, more than 130,000 American deaths could have been avoided.; had the U.S. matched Germany, the number would have been more than 215,000; had the U.S. matched its neighbor to the north, Canada, more than 266,000 deaths could have been avoided. Little wonder that Vermont Senator Bernie Sanders is a strong proponent of Canada's universal healthcare system.

One year after its first confirmed case of Covid-19, Joe Biden was inaugurated as America's 46th President. The contrast in leadership styles was dramatic. On the eve of his inauguration, along with Vice President-Elect Kamala Harris and their spouses, Biden held a memorial service at the Lincoln Memorial. 400 lights were illuminated along the edges of the Reflecting Pool, marking the more than 400,000 Americans who had died from Covid-19. During his Inaugural Address, President Biden asked for a moment of silent prayer, stating: *"We're entering what may be the toughest and deadliest period of the virus and must set aside politics and finally face this pandemic as one nation."*

Following the inauguration ceremony, he went to the Oval Office where his first three executive orders targeted Covid-19: requiring masks on federal property, rejoining the World Health Organization and establishing a White House Covid-19 response team led by Jeff Zients.

Biden signed a total of ten orders aimed at jump starting his national Covid-19 strategy to increase vaccinations and testing, lay the groundwork for reopening schools and businesses, and immediately increase the use of masks — including a requirement that Americans mask up for travel. Promising stringent adherence to public health guidance, Biden declared: *"To a nation waiting for action, let me be clear on this point: help is on the way."* When a reporter suggested that his goal of 100 million shots in his first 100 days in office is too low, Biden responded ""*When I announced it, you all said it's not possible. Come on, give me a break, man."* Dr. Fauci told reporters that if the vaccination campaign goes well, the U.S. could return to *"a degree of normality"* by the fall.

The 100 million shots goal was reached in 58 days; 200 million doses were administered during President Biden's first 100 days in office. Leading by example, President Biden wore a mask in public and he required his staff to do the same.

America should emulate the Scandinavians

FINLAND HAS BEEN THE world's happiest country for four years running; Denmark and Norway hold all but one of the other titles (World Happiness Report). The U.S. has yet to crack the top ten.

Among the 37 OECD member nations, four of the five Scandinavian countries are in the first quartile for lowest per capita fatality rates at August 31, 2021. They trail only the Pacific Rim countries (Australia, Japan, New Zealand and South Korea). Sweden was the outlier among the Scandinavian countries, ranking 22nd. All five countries have a robust public health infrastructure, sound social services safety nets and an abiding respect for science.

Their export-oriented economies are the envy of the European Union and, with low levels of debt as a percentage of GDP, they are well-positioned to spend their way out of the pandemic.

Early in the pandemic, Pulitzer Prize winning columnist Nicholas Kristof posed the question: *"Are female leaders better at fighting a pandemic?"*

Kristof compiled data from 21 countries, 13 led by men and 8 led by women. At that point in the pandemic, the fatality rate in male-led countries was six times higher than in the countries with female leaders. Kristof attributed the difference to male *"ego and bluster"* and contrasted it with the low-key, inclusive and evidence-based leadership in countries led by women.

Finland, Denmark, Norway and Iceland have women leaders. Sweden does not.

America should emulate the Scandinavians!

The Spanish flu pandemic of 1918-19 originated from a Kansas farm and spread globally, killing 675,000 Americans and as many as 50 million worldwide. On September 20, 2021, 20 months after its first confirmed case, America's Covid-19 death toll surpassed that of the worst pandemic in American history. With more effective early federal leadership in 2020, hundreds of thousands of Americans would still be alive today. The lessons learned from this pandemic must feed into the plans for any future pandemic to save American lives and to keep the nation's healthcare system functioning during difficult times.. America must use what has been learned to be much better prepared for any future national health emergency.

The Eichhorn – Hutchinson Allcare Plan for the United States

Appendix A summarizes the Eichhorn-Hutchinson Allcare Plan that is described in detail in Chapter 9 of "Healing American Healthcare, A Plan to Provide Care for All While Saving $1 Trillion a Year," written by Edward C. Eichhorn and Dr. Michael Hutchinson and published in 2019. To learn more about this plan read the complete chapter. The Eichhorn-Hutchinson Allcare Plan would require all employers to provide health insurance for their employees much like the German plan that began more than 100 years ago. Because choice is important to all Americans, this plan includes the option for private insurance as well as a public option based on Medicare. The healthcare market suffers from a general lack of competition. The public option that we envision will substantially reduce the cost of health insurance for employers and their employees if selected by employers to provide coverage for their employees.

This approach provides insurance companies with the opportunity to compete to retain their current clients' business, however they will have to develop programs that meet the price point of the new national public option. This much needed change to the market will do one of two things. It will spark innovation and creativity in the development of private health plans to compete with the public option or it will cause many of the insurers who lack the interest or ability to compete to leave this segment of the market. Either way employer healthcare costs will be drastically reduced, employee out-of-pocket costs will be reduced and virtually no one with a job will be uninsured or underinsured.

Over the years the health insurance industry has becomes a large segment of our national economy. As a national public insurance plan is introduced, the industry needs to have the opportunity to offer products to compete with a national health insurance plan. An employer could also elect to be self-insured, however in doing so they would have to meet the plan requirements of the public option.

The Allcare Plan would be very much like Medicare with several exceptions. Medicare Advantage would not be included in the plan for the public option. Medicare Advantage is approximately 30% of the annual cost of Medicare. It is the largest cost area for the program. This change would also provide insurance companies with an opportunity to offer Medicare Advantage-like plans to people who are under 65 and are not disabled. This would be a second market segment for private insurers to consider competing in that would be in addition to their offering health insurance plans that would compete with the new public plan. Today 60% of our employers provide coverage for more than 179 million Americans. While this change should be welcomed by employers who provide health insurance for their employees, employers who currently do not provide health insurance would have an increase in their overhead costs.

Other than eliminating the Medicare Advantage program from the coverage that would be offered in the public option plan, it would be the same as the rest of the Medicare Program. The new plan would also not include coverage for the disabled, especially those with kidney failure, ALS or other severe disabilities that qualify for Medicare today. These citizens with serious medical treatment needs would continue to be serviced by Medicare. This aspect of Medicare would remain unchanged.

As with Medicare, Part A of the new program would be for hospital coverage and the deductible would remain at $1,300 per year. Part B would still be for doctors' office visits with a 20% co-pay requirement. Part D would be for prescription coverage as it is today for Medicare. As previously stated, insurance companies could offer a Medicare Advantage type plan for people under 65. Medicare would remain largely unchanged; however, it would be able to negotiate drug prices for all its service segments. The plan would have no large deductibles as many of today's private insurance plans do. This major change will give subscribers the opportunity to seek care much earlier and should help to improve outcomes and lower the cost of treating serious illnesses because patients will have the opportunity to seek treatment much earlier in the disease process.

This new public health insurance plan would be a federal program; however, it would reduce the number of Americans who are on Medicaid because all employers would be obligated to provide health insurance. This change would reduce Medicaid funding in a significant way. It has been estimated that the Medicaid funding requirement would be reduced by at least 27% based on the number of workers who currently are eligible for Medicaid and work for employers who do not provide health insurance benefits for their employees. This savings would be shared by the Federal and State governments. Medicaid would remain as a safety net for the aged, the disabled and the unemployed poor.

Many authors have written about the lack of competition and the growth in bureaucracy and profits in the hospital, pharmaceutical and insurance industries. There are hundreds of insurance plans creating payment complexity that results in costly administrative waste and billing errors for hospital patients. The payment complexity can also create waste in the use of supplies for patient treatment. The fundamental idea of introducing a German-like health insurance plan is to create the completion that is missing from our market while reducing the cost of care by attacking excessive profit and bureaucratic waste. Our hospital, pharmaceutical and insurance industries are where most the costs (and profits) are that differentiate us from the rest of the world on a per capita basis. This is where the focus needs to be to begin the process of bringing our health care costs under control. The most important Allcare goal is to maintain or improve the quality of care in the United States while dramatically changing what it costs.

The four overall important objectives that if achieved would reduce the cost of healthcare in our economy over time by as much as $1 trillion per year while creating other positive economic impacts are:

1. Establish and provide a national healthcare option to compete with the private insurance industry in which all insurers are required to provide the same minimum benefits of the Medicare program.

2. Control drug costs through the establishment of a national negotiating platform that would be shared by all federal and state healthcare systems to prevent and eliminate price gouging in the pharmaceutical industry and unreasonable hospital mark ups of the drugs that they administer to their patients. The goal of this part of the plan is to reduce the per capita costs of our medications to match the per capita cost of other industrialized democracies that the United States is often compared to.

3. Reduce complexity by having a national standard on the cost of care: A national charge master for all services provided for patients at any hospital clinic or doctor's office anywhere in the United States regardless of the providers' tax status as for-profit or not-for-profile entities. Elimination of hospital facility fees for outpatient testing and standardizing all imaging and lab testing fees.

4. Use the healthcare data that is available to monitor costs, improve quality and reduce waste in the delivery of patient services and recommend that Accountable Care Organizations be provided with this data as they work to control costs and improve patient outcomes.

These important efforts to right size the cost of healthcare will not be easy. Almost every segment of the market will likely agree that the other segments of the industry will need to economize but their segment should be saved from cost reductions. Lobbyists will put forth many plausible strategies for their clients as to why they should be exempted from this effort to reduce our healthcare costs. In general, if this disruptive plan gains support, anyone who will be negatively impacted by these changes will be part of a huge outcry against any of these desperately needed changes. These changes if implemented would create incentives to compete for business in healthcare. While various current participants in the healthcare market may protest, the result would be no uninsured Americans, and lower healthcare costs for everyone. Even those who would protest this important change in our healthcare system will benefit. These four principles are worth fighting for. Fully implementing them in the U.S. economy could save $1 trillion per year.

Please review the infographic of the Eichhorn Hutchinson Allcare Plan on the following page that summarizes the plan's features and benefits.

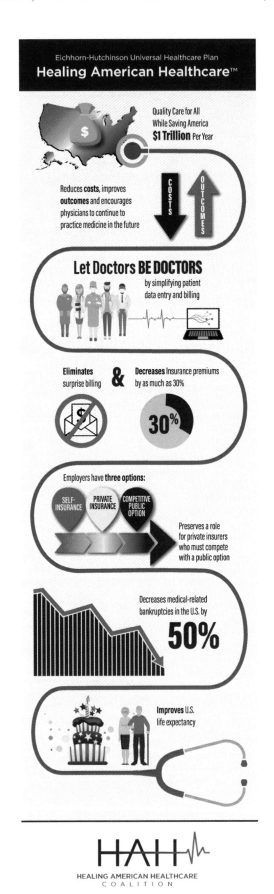

The Covid-19 Pandemic – How is the U.S. Doing?

This four-part series was written by co-author John Dalton for **GARDEN STATE FOCUS**, the award-winning quarterly news magazine of the New Jersey Chapter of the Healthcare Financial Management Association (HFMA). With more than 70,000 members, HFMA is the leading professional organization for individuals involved in healthcare finance. Mr. Dalton was the organization's 2001 recipient of its Individual Lifetime Achievement Award.

The COVID-19 Pandemic – How is the U.S. doing?

By John J. Dalton, FHFMA

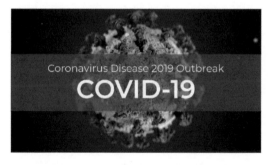

The COVID-19 pandemic has disrupted American lives like no event since the Spanish flu pandemic of 1918-19 that originated in Kansas and took 675,000 American lives and roughly 50 million lives worldwide. The SARS-CoV-2 virus is highly contagious, stealthy, insidious and potentially lethal, especially to older adults with multiple underlying conditions. First reported by China on December 31, 2019 after emerging in Wuhan, it rapidly spread throughout the world, with the first U.S. case confirmed on January 21, 2020.

Governmental responses to the threat varied widely, with some countries taking aggressive measures to prevent infection while others delayed action and resorted to implementing mitigation measures to "flatten the curve." As I write today, the world is four months into the greatest public health threat in more than a century, the federal government's "Stay at Home" order is expiring and at least 58,500 Americans have died during April alone, more than the 58,220 who perished during the entire Vietnam War. In comparison, the eight month 2017-18 flu season was the worst in the past 10 years killing an estimated 61,000 Americans.

Here at the epicenter of America's epidemic, hospital ICUs have been overwhelmed as the disease ravaged the New York Metro area. Many more months will pass before judgments can be made on how well or poorly various countries dealt with the pandemic, but some evidence already is emerging.

As a metrics-driven engineer deprived of the distractions of playing golf and watching Yankee baseball, I have instead been monitoring COVID-19 data from several sources while sheltering in place. The COVID-19 daily updates have reported on data elements that include tests conducted, cases confirmed, positivity rates, ICU beds and ventilator needs, and the numbers of patient deaths and recoveries. Some calculate a raw fatality rate (% of deaths/# of confirmed cases) as an indicator, but that has significant limitations. The number of confirmed cases depends on the extent of each country's testing program and the scope varies widely. The author believes that the most important key performance indicator (KPI) of a country's effectiveness in combating the pandemic will be an outcome measure - the fatality rate per 100,000 residents.

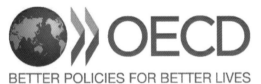

Using COVID-19 data from the World Health Organization (WHO), I focused on the performance of the 37 member countries of the Organisation for Economic Co-operation and Development (OECD) as of April 30. With a total population of 1.3 billion, the 37 OECD member nations had recorded 200,646 fatalities. Chart 1 illustrates the current results for 20 of the member countries. Data for all 37 countries are contained in Table 2 - COVID-19 Confirmed Cases and Fatalities, 4/30/2020 following the article.

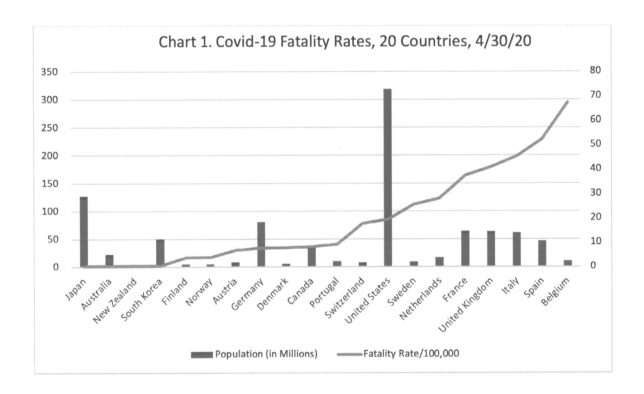

The range of results among the world's most developed economies is shocking. Four countries (Australia, Japan, Korea and New Zealand) were able to stop the virus in its tracks with fewer than one death per 100,000 residents. At the other extreme, five European countries (Belgium, France, Italy, Spain and the United Kingdom) are experiencing fatality rates of more than 30 deaths per 100,000 residents. With a current fatality rate of 19.4 deaths per 100,000 residents, the U.S. sits in 29th place. Were I a college professor grading on a curve, America would receive a "C-" grade. Among the largest Western Europe nations, only Germany earns a "B" grade at 7.8 per 100,000. With fatality rates per 1,000 ranging from 37.5 to 52.2 per 100,000 residents, France, Italy, Spain and the United Kingdom are at the bottom of the barrel.

Public health experts, doctoral candidates and Congressional Committees will spend the next several years conducting post-mortem dissections of the COVID-19 pandemic. I will leave the second-guessing to them and limit my comments to four countries that earned an "A" grade and the U.S. response, then discuss briefly about what the new normal might look like.

Lessons from the "A" Nations

AMONG THE OECD's 37 member nations, densely populated Japan and Korea and sparsely populated Australia and New Zealand clearly stand at the head of the class. Why were these four countries, with differing cultures and governance, able to prevent COVID-19 from reaching epidemic proportions? Did Japan and Korea's proximity to China and their Oriental culture play a role? Did Australia and New Zealand's location in the Southern Hemisphere where it was summer affect their results?

Korea's first confirmed COVID-19 case on January 21 coincided with the U.S.'s first case. How did this country of 50.4 million succeed in quickly flattening the curve? The key steps taken were intervene fast, before it's a crisis; test early, often and safely; implement contact tracing, isolation and surveillance; and enlist the public's help. Its highest daily new cases occurred on 2/29 and have been dropping since.

In protecting its 127.3 million residents, Japan acted quickly to prevent an influx of cases from overseas. On February 3, it barred the entry of people who had a history of traveling to Hubei province, or Chinese nationals with a Hubei province-issued passport. A month later, the entry restrictions were expanded to include people from certain regions of South Korea, Italy, and Iran as well as two-week quarantines for all visitors coming from China and South Korea. Japan's central policy has been to focus on providing medical attention to those who are severely ill in order to prevent the nation's health care infrastructure from becoming overwhelmed, and to do extensive contact tracing to identify infection clusters.

With fewer ICU beds per capita than hard-hit Italy, New Zealand had to act decisively and fast after its first case of coronavirus was confirmed on February 28. Prime Minister Jacinta Ardern announced on March 14 that anyone entering the country would need to self-isolate for two weeks, then on March 19 banned foreigners from entering the country. On March 23, when Ardern announced that the country of 4.5 million was going into lockdown, there were 102 confirmed cases -- and no deaths. Since April 1, there has been only one new confirmed case.

Following global criticism of his handling of Australia's wildfires last Fall, Prime Minister Scott Morrison's response to the pandemic has largely centered on shutting its borders, limiting public gatherings and conducting large-scale testing and contact tracing. Social gatherings of more than two people were also forbidden and leaving the house is permitted only for essential reasons like buying food and exercising. Travelling overseas is banned, foreigners are not allowed to enter the country, and Australians who return from other countries are kept in mandatory quarantine at specially designated hotels for two weeks. Australia also launched an app to track COVID-19 cases among its 23.5 million residents that may help to speed up the process of easing social distancing measures.

How Do U.S. Results Stack Up?

For once, the U.S. is not at the bottom of the barrel among OECD member nations. At 19.4 fatalities per 100,000 residents, the U.S. is 29th out of the 37 OECD member nations compared with the OECD average of 15.3 fatalities per 100,000 residents.

Four years ago, I wrote a series of articles, *"American Healthcare: Worst Value in the Developed World?"* that examined the following paradox: America has the best-equipped hospitals and most thoroughly trained physicians in the world, spends a higher percentage of GDP on healthcare, yet according to the Commonwealth Fund, delivers "High cost care of mediocre quality." The articles compared 22 OECD member countries with differing approaches to universal healthcare and found that, in the aggregate, countries with government funded single payer systems produced the best outcomes on four key health indicators: life expectancy at birth, both sexes, infant mortality rate, child mortality rate and adult mortality rate.

Next, the series moved on to compare the U.S. with three major industrialized countries with characteristics similar to the United States – Germany, France and the United Kingdom (UK) – to explore some of the underlying reasons for the disparity between America and its OECD counterparts. Table 1, below, displays healthcare spending and key health indicators for the four countries.

Table 1 - Healthcare Spending and Key Health Indicators, France, Germany, UK and U.S.

Healthcare % of GDP - 2013 (2)	Health Spending per Capita, 2011 (3)	Country	Type of Universal Health Care (1)	Life Expectancy @ Birth, both sexes 2012 (4)	Infant Mortality Rate per 1000, 2012 (4)	Child Mortality Rate, per 1000, 2012 (4)
10.9	$4,111	France	Two-Tier	82	3	4
11.0	$4,495	Germany	Insurance Mandate	81	3	4
8.5	$3,405	United Kingdom	Single Payer	81	4	5
16.4	$8,508	United States	None	79	6	7

1. Modern Healthcare, February 8, 2016, p. 34
2. OECD Health Statistics, 2015, FOCUS. on Health Spending, July 2015
3. Commonwealth Fund, 2014, "Mirror, Mirror on the Wall: How the U.S. Health Care System Compares Internationally"
4. World Health Statistics, 2014, PART III, Global Health Indicators, WHO

With the best-equipped hospitals and most thoroughly trained physicians in the world, America excels at treating and curing illnesses. However, it lacks the robust commitment to public health and prevention of France, Germany and the UK. Despite that commitment, France and the UK have not fared well during the stress test of the global pandemic with fatality rates per 100,000 of 37.5 and 41.0, respectively. Germany has fared far better at 7.8 per 100,000.

How has Germany done so well? In her 4/4/20 article in the New York Times (A German Exception? Why the Country's Coronavirus Death Rate Is Low), Katrin Bennhold asserted that a key reason for the low fatality rate is that Germany has been testing far more people, catching many with few or no symptoms. Charité Hospital in Berlin developed a test mid-January, posted the formula online and laboratories throughout the country built up a stock of test kits. Germany's public health system has 34 ICU beds per 100,000 residents, more than double the OECD average of 15.9, so surge capacity was not an issue.

Germany has had universal healthcare since 1883 and achieved full interoperability in 2008. Medical insurance is mandatory, and Germans can choose from more than 100 not-for profit insurance plans. There is a government buy-in for low income and unemployed. However, to many, the "secret sauce" in Germany's low mortality rate has been the leadership of Chancellor Angela Merkel, a scientist by training, who has communicated clearly, calmly and regularly throughout the crisis. Prof. Hans-Georg Kräusslich, head of virology at University Hospital in Heidelberg, summed it up: *"Maybe our biggest strength in Germany is the rational decision-making at the highest level of government combined with the trust the government enjoys in the population."*

Although well behind Germany's fatality rate, the U.S. has produced better results than France or the UK thus far. In his 4/1/20 BBC News article (Coronavirus: Things the US has got wrong - and got right), Anthony Zurcher first cited the following mistakes:

- Testing delays due to the administration's disregard of pandemic response plans and failure to staff its public health bureaucracy;
- Medical supply shortages (masks, gloves, gowns and ventilators) due both to the government's failure to maintain the stockpile and failure to move quickly when the crisis became apparent;
- Messaging "whiplash" and political squabbles, downplaying the threat during January and February; and
- Social distancing failures like the packed Florida beaches during spring break.

On a more positive note, Zurcher cited strong state leadership with many governors "taking decisive early steps to close schools and issue shelter in place orders." He also cited America's research firepower and its ability to devise new strategies to defeat the pandemic including rapid-response tests, vaccine development and treatment options. Although swamped by the pandemic surge, the New York Metro healthcare industry has been learning on the fly. Successes to date include development of the Rutgers Saliva Test for the SARS-CoV-2 virus that received emergency use authorization from the FDA on 4/13. Using easy-to-collect saliva samples instead of the more difficult deep nose swabs reduces the need for health care workers to wear and discard precious gowns and masks.

Other promising developments include the use of convalescent plasma (CP) therapy in severe COVID-19 patients and, most recently, preliminary data showing that remdesivir speeds up the recovery of some COVID-19 patients: median time to recovery was 11 days for patients treated with remdesivir compared with 15 days for those who received placebo.

Other efforts are identifying which symptomatic patients are more likely to progress to acute respiratory distress syndrome (ARDS) a type of lung failure identified in the 2003 outbreak of the SARS coronavirus. Many patients seeking treatment are in worse shape than they realize. Their blood oxygen saturation levels are exceedingly low although they are hardly gasping for breath, a condition known as "silent hypoxia." Home use of a pulse oximeter can detect lower blood saturation levels so that treatment can begin earlier.

The COVID-19 pandemic is neither a sprint nor a marathon, but an ultra-marathon. Fatality rates per 100,000 residents will continue to rise until an effective vaccine is developed and enough doses administered to attain herd immunity to the SARS-CoV-2 virus. Until then, I am confident that the combination of the world's best equipped hospitals and most thoroughly trained physicians will continue to minimize the number of American deaths resulting from this insidious virus.

Table 2 – COVID-19 Confirmed Cases and Fatalities, 4/30/2020

Confirmed Cases (1)	Fatalities (1)	Fatality Rate (%)	37 OECD Countries	Population (2)	Cases per 100,000	Fatalities per 100,000
14,088	415	2.9%	Japan	127,298,000	11.1	0.3
6,746	90	1.3%	Australia	23,491,000	28.7	0.4
1,391	22	1.6%	Slovak Republic	5,415,949	25.7	0.4
1,129	19	1.7%	New Zealand	4,509,000	25.0	0.4
10,765	247	2.3%	South Korea	50,423,000	21.3	0.5
5,949	269	4.5%	Colombia	49,650,000	12.0	0.5
849	15	1.8%	Latvia	1,920,000	44.2	0.8
14,885	216	1.5%	Chile	17,556,820	84.8	1.2
2,576	139	5.4%	Greece	11,090,000	23.2	1.3
16,752	1,569	9.4%	Mexico	118,395,100	14.1	1.3
1,375	45	3.3%	Lithuania	2,794,329	49.2	1.6
12,640	624	4.9%	Poland	38,533,790	32.8	1.6
7,579	227	3.0%	Czech Republic	10,524,820	72.0	2.2
2,775	312	11.2%	Hungary	9,886,774	28.1	3.2
1,797	10	0.6%	Iceland	310,013	579.7	3.2
4,906	206	4.2%	Finland	5,440,000	90.2	3.8
1,666	50	3.0%	Estonia	1,320,174	126.2	3.8
7,667	202	2.6%	Norway	5,137,000	149.3	3.9
117,589	3,081	2.6%	Turkey	76,054,620	154.6	4.1
1,418	89	6.3%	Slovenia	2,061,623	68.8	4.3
15,782	212	1.3%	Israel	4,609,600	342.4	4.6
15,364	580	3.8%	Austria	8,468,570	181.4	6.8
159,119	6,288	4.0%	Germany	80,645,810	197.3	7.8
9,008	443	4.9%	Denmark	5,614,932	160.4	7.9
50,363	2,904	5.8%	Canada	34,880,490	144.4	8.3
24,505	973	4.0%	Portugal	10,457,300	234.3	9.3
3,769	89	2.4%	Luxembourg	530,946	709.9	16.8
29,324	1,407	4.8%	Switzerland	7,912,398	370.6	17.8
1,062,492	61,931	5.8%	United States	318,857,000	333.2	19.4
20,302	2,462	12.1%	Sweden	9,609,000	211.3	25.6
20,253	1,190	5.9%	Ireland	4,609,000	439.4	25.8
38,802	4,711	12.1%	Netherlands	16,804,430	230.9	28.0
127,066	24,054	18.9%	France	64,062,000	198.3	37.5
165,225	26,097	15.8%	United Kingdom	63,650,000	259.6	41.0
203,591	27,682	13.6%	Italy	61,178,360	332.8	45.2
212,917	24,275	11.4%	Spain	46,464,000	458.2	52.2
47,859	7,501	15.7%	Belgium	11,128,250	430.1	67.4
2,440,283	200,646	8.2%	Total OECD	1,311,294,098	186.1	15.3
3,235,276	229,669	7.1%	Global Total			

DATA SOURCES: 1. World Health Organization, CDC
2. Organisation for Economic Co-operation and Development

The COVID-19 Pandemic – How is the U.S. doing? Part 2

By John J. Dalton, FHFMA

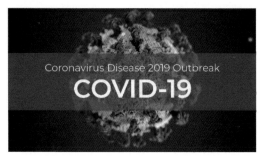

THE SHORT ANSWER – not well.

In the article written May 1st that appeared in the Spring issue, I had laid out the case for monitoring per capita fatality rates as the key performance indicator (KPI) for initially assessing a country's performance in responding to the global pandemic, then compared America's performance with the other member countries of the Organisation for Economic Co-operation and Development (OECD) as of April 30 (1). With 61,931 deaths and a fatality rate of 19.4/100,000 residents, the U.S. ranked 29th among the 37 OECD members.

As I complete this article on September 21st, eight months after the U.S.'s first confirmed Covid-19 case in Washington state, more than 200,000 Americans have perished and the U.S. has slipped to 33rd place in the OECD, trailed only by Spain, Chile, the United Kingdom (UK) and Belgium (see Table 1 - Confirmed Cases and Fatality Rates, OECD Countries as of 9/20/2020). Spain's initial outbreak was in Madrid, its capital, business and international hub, and had a second surge in August after loosening restrictions (2). Chile was hit by the pandemic in June. Its limited testing capacity and slow turnaround times amplified the impact that was further exacerbated by the government's lack of transparency in reporting infection rates (3). The UK's initial approach of reaching "herd immunity" allowed community spread that has resulted in a per capita fatality rate of 65.5/100,000 (4). Belgium's failure to protect its nursing home residents is tragic, accounting for roughly 58% of the country's fatalities, a much higher percentage than in other developed countries (5).

Conversely, three of the top five countries at April 30 continue to lead the OECD (New Zealand, Korea and Japan) while Australia has slipped in the rankings due to a severe outbreak in Melbourne, the country's second largest city (6,7). The earlier article described the measures taken by each of the four to control the pandemic. With the lowest per capita death rate in Europe, the Slovak Republic was the other country in the in the top five (8). Initially caught unaware, the government's decision to institute a national lockdown effective March 16, 10 days after the country confirmed its first coronavirus case, was highly effective. It included closing all schools, restaurants, bars, and shops except for grocery stores, pharmacies, and banks, banned all public events and gatherings, closed airports and quarantined citizens returning from abroad. Its residents immediate and universal compliance has resulted in Europe's lowest per capita fatality rate of 0.72/100,000 (see Chart 1, Covid-19 Fatality Rates, 20 OECD Countries).

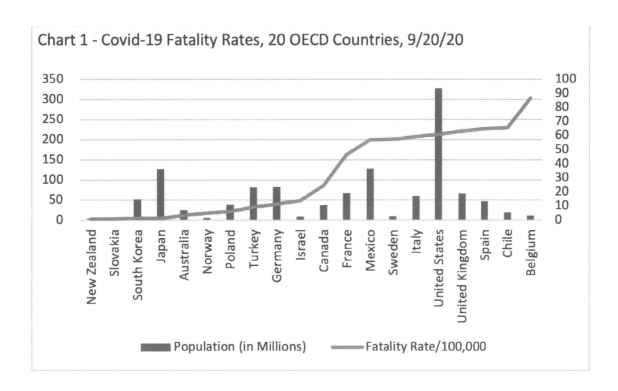

Chart 1 - Covid-19 Fatality Rates, 20 OECD Countries, 9/20/20

The U.S. fatality rate of 60.9/100,000 is nearly 60% higher than the OECD average of 37.8/100,000. Had the U.S. merely matched the OECD average, more than 75,000 Americans would be alive today. Had we matched the performance of Canada, our neighbor to the north, nearly 120,000 more Americans would be alive today. Hindsight is 20/20 and there has been and will continue to be a lot of Monday morning quarterbacking.

The first U.S. case was diagnosed in Washington state January 20, and subsequently determined to be the D614 strain of the novel coronavirus. The more virulent G614 strain hit the Metro New York area, the global epicenter of the pandemic during March and April. New Jersey was hardest hit, with 16,046 deaths and a fatality rate of 180.7/100,000, trailed slightly by New York state with 33,081 deaths and a fatality rate of 170.1/100,000 (see Chart 2 - Covid-19 Fatality Rates, 20 Selected States, 9/20/20). New York City has had 23,771 deaths for a fatality rate of 283/100,000, more than three times Belgium's 86.8/100,000 fatality rate.

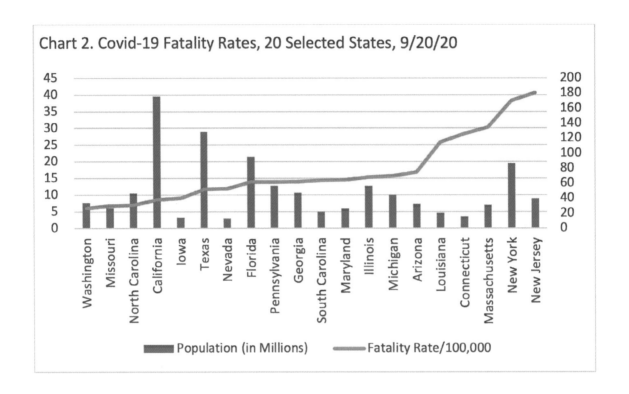

This article will focus first on what we've learned about COVID-19 during the past four months, next discuss key factors that have determined whether a country has succeeded in controlling the pandemic, then conclude with an update on progress towards a safe effective vaccine.

What Have We Learned about Covid-19?

EARLY ON WE LEARNED that the SARS-CoV-2 virus is highly contagious, stealthy, insidious and potentially lethal, especially to adults over 65 with multiple underlying conditions. Initial guidance included wearing masks, social distancing, frequent hand washing and sanitizing of high-touch surfaces. As the global pandemic continued to rage through the summer months, research studies in several countries provided much-needed insights into how Covid-19 is contracted and who is more likely to contract it. Some key findings include:

- Airborne transmission is the most dominant route for the spread of Covid-19;
- Loss of the sense of smell is a key indicator of infection;
- Covid-19 hits men harder than women;
- Communities of color are more likely to be vulnerable to infection;
- Obese individuals who contract Covid-19 are more likely to be hospitalized;
- For severe cases where hospitalization is required, where one is treated matters;
- Even in less severe cases, Covid-19's lingering effects are of concern; and

• A supercomputer analysis of more than 2.5 billion genetic combinations has provided a model - the bradykinin hypothesis - that explains many of Covid-19's bizarre symptoms.

Masks Must Be Mandatory. In June, the National Academy of Sciences published a research paper identifying airborne transmission as the most dominant route for the spread of Covid-19 (9). The authors studied the transmission pathways of the coronavirus by evaluating the trend and comparative mitigation efforts in the three first epicenters including Wuhan China, Italy and New York City. They found that that airborne transmission of the virus represents the most likely route to community spread of the disease. When considering the mitigation strategies of safe distancing, avoiding large gatherings and wearing a protective mask when in public, they found that the most significant mitigation factor to reducing the spread of the virus was mandating face coverings. From April 6 to May 9 this practice reduced infections by 78,000 in Italy and by over 66,000 from April 17 to May 9 in New York City.

Understanding the scientific basis for airborne transmission of this respiratory virus should dictate public policy to flatten the infection curve in the cities and states where hot spots are evolving. The research paper does not minimize the importance of all mitigation strategies to control the spread of Covid-19. However, these measures were started in Italy and New York City well before mandating face coverings. Wuhan China implemented all of the mitigation practices as well as extensive testing and contact tracing which lowered their infection curve more rapidly when compared with the other two epicenters.

A study published in the June issue of Health Affairs provides direct evidence on the effects of state government mandates in the U.S. for face mask use in public issued by 15 states plus DC between April 8 and May 15 (10). It estimated that as many as 230,000–450,000 Covid-19 cases may have been averted based on when states passed these mandates. The authors concluded: *As countries worldwide and states begin to relax social distancing restrictions and considering the high likelihood of a second Covid-19 wave in the fall/winter, requiring use of face masks in public might help in reducing Covid-19 spread.*

These studies - and others - make it clear that policy makers and political leaders throughout the U.S. need to be aware of and respect the science behind the community spread of Covid-19. Covid-19 is not political, infecting Democrats, Republicans and Independents alike. Mask wearing must be made mandatory until a safe, effective vaccine is developed and a significant percentage of the most vulnerable Americans have received it.

Anosmia = Infected. Think you're infected by Covid-19? Your nose knows! At least half of confirmed cases worldwide had anosmia (loss of smell); in Germany, it was more than 2/3rds. An Iranian study found that 59 of 60 patients exhibited various smell dysfunctions (11). Harvard professor of immunology Andrew Chan, co-founder of the Covid Symptom Study, concludes that the strongest predictor of a Covid-19 infection is a loss of taste or smell, a symptom that is relatively uncommon in other viral syndromes (12). Decreased smell function is a major marker for the SARS-CoV-2 infection. Smell testing should be used for early identification of Covid-19 patients in need of early treatment or quarantine.

Gender Matters. Covid-19 infects men at a higher rate and men have more difficult outcomes than women. Dr. Akiko Iwasaki, Professor of Immunology and Molecular Biology at the Howard Hughes Medical school at Yale University, led a research team that examined how men and women's immune systems respond to this virus infection (13). The researchers found that men develop higher cytokine levels and women generally develop higher

T-cell levels as an early response. The cytokine reaction can cause an inflammation that attacks the virus in the lungs but also results in reduced oxygen levels and fluid buildup that can cause other organs to fail. T-cells are white blood cells that attach to viruses.

Older men do not develop T-cell responses as well as younger people. Older women can also develop higher cytokine reactions and therefore can have worse outcomes than other women who do not. Dr. Iwasaki has said these findings *"suggest we need different strategies to ensure that treatments and vaccines are equally effective for both men and women."* Dr. Amesh Adalja, an infectious disease expert at Johns Hopkins University commented, *"We are increasingly seeing that a one-size-fits-all strategy is not always possible, and precision medicine -- based on each individual's unique characteristics -- is likely the best approach."* Clearly, a basic understanding of how the immune system responds to this virus based on both sex and age is crucial to learning how care givers can produce better outcomes in treating Covid–19.

Communities of Color Were Hit Harder. NPR recently analyzed Covid-19 demographic data collected by the Covid Racial Tracker, a joint project of the Antiracist Research & Policy Center and the Covid Tracking Project (14). The review found finds that in 32 states plus Washington D.C., African-Americans are dying at rates higher than their proportion of the population. In 21 states, it's substantially higher, more than 50% above what would be expected. Likewise, Latinos and Hispanics test positive for the coronavirus at rates higher than would be expected for their share of the population in all but one of the 44 jurisdictions that report Hispanic ethnicity data (42 states plus Washington D.C.). The rates are two times higher in 30 states, and over four times higher in eight states.

African-Americans have higher rates of underlying conditions, including diabetes, heart disease, and lung disease, that are linked to more severe cases of Covid-19. Both African-Americans and Latinos are over-represented in low wage essential jobs that increase their exposure to the virus. In addition, dense, multi-generational housing conditions makes it easier for the virus to spread in Latino communities. Given the pandemic's disparate toll on communities of color, in particular low-income ones, the public health response should include helping to meet basic needs like providing food, wage supports and even temporary housing for people who get sick or exposed to the virus.

BMI>40? Beware of Covid-19! There's some evidence that obesity itself can increase the likelihood of serious complications from a coronavirus infection (15). One study of more than 5,200 infected people, including 35% who were obese, found that the chances of hospitalization rose for people with higher BMIs, even when considering other conditions that could put them at risk. The increased risk for serious Covid-19 illness appears more pronounced with extreme obesity, or a BMI of 40 or higher. Multiple factors make it more difficult for obese individuals to fight the coronavirus, including chronic inflammation and how fat is distributed in the body.

Place of Treatment Matters. JAMA Internal Medicine recently published a large study that examined mortality rates for more than 2,200 critically ill coronavirus patients in 65 hospitals throughout the country and found that patients admitted to hospitals with fewer than 50 ICU beds were three times more likely to die (16). An earlier investigative piece in the New York Times found that at the peak of the pandemic, patients at some community hospitals were three times more likely to die than patients in medical centers in wealthier areas (17).

Covid-19'S Lingering Effects. Evidence is mounting that many Covid-19 survivors face months and possibly longer periods of debilitating complications. Symptoms include breathing difficulties, neurological issues, heart complications, kidney disease and motor skill problems. Some hard-hit countries - including the United States, Britain and Italy - are considering whether these long-term effects can be considered a "post-Covid syndrome." Dr. Bruce Lee of the City University of New York, Public School of Health estimates that if 20% of the U.S. population contracts this virus, the one-year cost could be $50 billion (18).

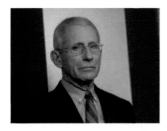

Like other viruses, Covid-19's effects often will linger long after the initial encounter, even among younger patients with mild symptoms. Dr. Gregory Poland, a Covid-19 expert at the Mayo Clinic warns that some of the possible long-term effects can affect even patients who are asymptomatic or have mild cases: *"I think it's an argument for why we take this disease so seriously."*(19) He added *"we're going to need to study those as vigorously as we did the acute symptoms."* Mount Sinai will lead a multi-center trial that includes monitoring patients who suffered acute kidney injury while hospitalized (20). Dr. Anthony Fauci, Director of the National Institute of Allergy and Infectious Diseases since 1984, said post-viral Covid-19 syndrome is fast becoming a patient care problem: *"Brain fog, fatigue and difficulty in concentrating, so this is something we really need to seriously look at."* (21)

A Eureka Moment? At Oak Ridge National Labs, site of the world's second fastest supercomputer (and World War Two's Manhattan Project), scientists crunched data on more than 40,000 genes from 17,000 genetic samples analyzing 2.5 billion genetic combinations (22). It took more than a week, leading to the bradykinin hypothesis that provides a model that explains many of Covid-19's bizarre symptoms. It also suggests more than ten potential treatments, including some that are FDA approved. Generally, a Covid-19 infection begins when the virus enters the body through ACE2 receptors in the nose, then proceeds through the body entering cells where ACE2 also is present. Its insidious progression is well documented in this study. The bradykinin hypothesis provides a unified theory for how Covid-19 works. Dr. Daniel Jacobson, lead researcher is clear: *"We have to get this message out."*

What Are the Keys to Success?

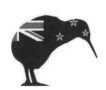

COUNTRIES RESPONSES TO THE global pandemic have varied broadly, with some noteworthy successes as well as many dismal failures. Faced with fewer ICU beds per capita than hard-hit Italy, New Zealand had to act decisively after its first coronavirus case was confirmed February 28 (6). On March 14 Prime Minister Ardern imposed a two-week self-isolation period on anyone entering the country; on March 19 she banned foreigners from entering the country; and on March 23 locked down the country of 4.9 million. It worked - New Zealand continues to lead the OECD with the lowest fatality rate in the developed world. Similarly, Korea's first Covid-19 case was confirmed the same day as the US (7). However, Korea acted quickly to "flatten the curve" by intervening fast, before it's a crisis, testing early, often and safely; implementing contact tracing, isolation and surveillance; and enlisting the public's help.

Among the major Western democracies, only Germany has succeeded in keeping its fatality rate below the OECD average (23). One key reason is that Germany has been testing far more people, catching many with few or no symptoms. Charité Hospital in Berlin developed a test mid-January, posted the formula online and laboratories throughout the country built up a stock of test kits. Germany also has aggressively tracked contacts and practiced social distancing, copying Korea's strategy. Germany's robust public health system had 28,000 intensive care beds equipped with ventilators (34 per 100,000 people) compared with 12 per 100,000 in Italy and has added capacity since the outbreak.

To many, the "secret sauce" in Germany's low mortality rate has been the leadership of Chancellor Angela Merkel, a scientist by training, who has communicated clearly, calmly and regularly throughout the crisis. Prof. Hans-Georg Kräusslich, head of virology at University Hospital in Heidelberg, summed it up: *"Maybe our biggest strength in Germany is the rational decision-making at the highest level of government combined with the trust the government enjoys in the population."*

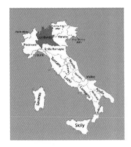

At the other end of the spectrum, northern Italy was hit hard, especially in Lombardy (24). With 1/6th of Italy's 60 million people, it's the most densely populated region, home to the business capital in Milan and Italy's industrial heartland, accounting for 21% of GDP. With the country's highest percentage over 65, Lombardy also has 20% of Italy's nursing homes. When Italy became the first European country to halt air travel from China on January 31, it was already too late. Doctors treating patients for pneumonia didn't know it was Covid-19 and were unprepared for many patients rapid decline in the ability to breathe. After years of budget cuts, Italy has only 8.6 ICU beds per 100,000 people, well below the OECD average of 15.9, so many PCPs were treating patients at home, some with supplemental oxygen. Testing was limited by inadequate lab capacity, so PCPs didn't know whether they or their patients were infected. PPE was in short supply and inadequate. A blistering April 7 letter from the doctors' association to regional authorities listed seven errors in their handling of the crisis.

The region's industrial lobbying group resisted shutting down production until March 26, long after Rome's March 7 shut down order. Lombardy's nursing homes house more than 24,000 elderly; of 3,045 deaths from February 2 to April 15, 1,625 were either positive for the virus or showed symptoms. A March 30 regional decree directed nursing homes to not hospitalize sick residents over 75 if they had other health problems. Some nursing homes refused to let staff wear masks to avoid frightening patients. Some local authorities threatened loss of accreditation if the nursing home refused to allow visitors. The rest of the country learned from Lombardy and now has a lower fatality rate than the US.

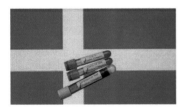

Sweden initially assumed that the Coronavirus was like the seasonal flu and took a light touch approach to controlling its spread. With a fatality rate much higher than its Scandinavian neighbors, Anders Tegnell, Sweden's chief epidemiologist, admitted in a June radio interview that there was *"quite obviously a potential for improvement in what we have done"* in Sweden (25). Tegnell had previously been critical of other countries' strict lockdowns as unsustainable in the long run. Sweden closed schools for all over-16s and banned gatherings of more than 50, but shops, restaurants and gyms remained open. Prime Minister Stefan Lovfen defended Sweden's approach as just about right but noted that it had failed to protect care homes where half of all Sweden's Covid-19 deaths have occurred.

With the highest fatality rate in the OECD, Belgium still defends its failed approach (5). Although hospital ICU beds were available throughout the peak period, hospitals and paramedics sometimes denied care to elderly people. When the pandemic hit northern Italy in February, Maggie De Block, Belgium's federal health minister, played down the risk: *"It isn't a very aggressive virus. You would have to sneeze in someone's face to pass it on,"* adding *"If the temperature rises, it will probably disappear."*

Although government reports had recommended infectious-disease training for nursing home doctors, public help in stockpiling PPE, and including nursing homes in the national pandemic plan, the proposals went nowhere. Belgian bureaucracy exacerbated the response: it has nine health ministers who answer to six parliaments. Testing capacity was limited with hospitals taking priority. When nursing home testing finally began April 8 (after more than 2,000 residents already had died), 20% tested positive. At the outbreak's peak only 14% of gravely ill residents were admitted to hospitals according to data compiled by Belgian scientists. The rest were left to receive palliative care. According to University of Antwerp professor Niel Hens, 1,100 of the nation's 2,400 intensive care beds were free at the peak of the pandemic. Ms. De Block has defended the government response stating, *"Careful counting, not mismanagement, explains the country's death toll,"* noting with pride that Belgium never ran out of hospital beds. Its failure to protect its nursing home residents is tragic, accounting for roughly 58% of the country's fatalities, a much higher percentage than in other developed countries.

The Foundation for Research on Equal Opportunity conducted an in-depth review of per capita fatality rates in 31 high income countries through mid-August, including four that are not OECD members (Hong Kong, Singapore, Taiwan, United Arab Emirates) (26). The review considered variables including stringency of economic restrictions, relative isolation and type of universal healthcare. It found no correlation between the format of a country's health insurance system and its ranking. Among countries with single payer systems, Australia fared well, but Italy, Spain and the UK did not. Countries with private insurance and/or consumer-driven models are also all over the rankings.

Overall, five Pacific Rim countries (Hong Kong, Korea, Japan, Singapore, Taiwan, and New Zealand) nations fared the best in the review's Pandemic Performance rankings. Except for Germany, the major Western democracies (France, Italy, Spain, the UK and the US) did not. A key factor in successfully controlling Covid-19 was SARS "muscle memory." Residents of these countries were acutely aware of the threat posed by Covid-19 due to their prior experience with the SARS-CoV pandemic in 2002-03. Asian governments took the threat more seriously early on, and enacted aggressive contact tracing measures and had already built up stockpiles of personal protective equipment.

In his New York Times article, Pulitzer Prize winning columnist Nicholas Kristof posed the question: *"Are female leaders better at fighting a pandemic?"* Kristof compiled data from 21 countries, 13 led by men and 8 led by women (27). The Covid-19 fatality rate was 214 per million in male-led countries and 36 per million in female-led countries including Denmark, Finland, Germany, Iceland, New Zealand, Norway and Taiwan. Residents of the 13 male-led countries were six times more likely to die from Covid-19 than residents of the 8 female-led countries. Noting that *"Virtually every country that has experienced coronavirus mortality at a rate of more than 150 per million inhabitants is male-led,"* Kristof attributes the difference to male *"ego and bluster"* and contrasts it with the low-key, inclusive and evidence-based leadership in countries led by women.

A Safe Effective Vaccine – When?

EARLY ON, ANTHONY ZURCHER, the BBC's North American reporter, wrote about what the US had gotten wrong, and what it got right (28). He criticized testing delays due to the administration's disregard of pandemic response plans and failure to staff its public health bureaucracy; medical supply shortages due both to the government's failure to maintain the stockpile and failure to move quickly when the crisis became apparent; messaging "whiplash" and political squabbles, downplaying the threat; and social distancing failures like the packed Florida beaches during spring break. Other flaws cited include high costs, a lack of universal coverage and supply chains unable to withstand a shock.

On the other hand, Zurcher expressed optimism that America's research firepower, with medical researchers and drug companies rushing to learn more about the virus and devise new strategies to defeat the pandemic including rapid-response tests, vaccine development and treatment options will help the US to recover.

At this juncture, global knowledge about the disease, its diagnosis progression and treatment has grown exponentially. With more rapid and extensive testing and better treatment, the OECD's case fatality rate has dropped from 7.1% on May 1st to 4.2% today – still far higher than the seasonal flu. At 2.9%, the U.S. case fatality rate is half the 5.8% on May 1st (see Table 1). Remdesevir and dexamethasome have shown promise in reducing Covid-19's severity, while much more needs to be learned about its lingering effects.

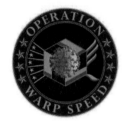 Operation Warp Speed (OWS) is a public–private partnership, initiated by the Trump administration, to facilitate and accelerate the development, manufacturing, and distribution of Covid-19 vaccines, therapeutics, and diagnostics (29). It ranks as one of the most ambitious scientific endeavors in modern U.S. history. If all goes well, the fast-tracking of vaccine development, which normally takes years, will have been telescoped down to about a year. To date, the fastest a vaccine was ever developed was four years. OWS has already spent over $10 billion to help vaccine makers to build out production capacity before knowing whether their vaccine is safe and effective.

The theory is that, if a vaccine is proven to be safe and effective, it can immediately be deployed. Contracts with six manufacturers already are in place. Three of them - AstraZeneca, Moderna, and Pfizer — have vaccines that generated immune responses without causing serious side effects and have initiated phase 3 clinical trials, enrolling 30,000 volunteers (30). OWS Chief Advisor Moncef Slaoui said that it was *"extremely unlikely but not impossible"* for those trials to finish by the end of October. A more realistic estimate is that a vaccine will become available for high-risk populations by the end of 2020. The CEOs of nine pharmaceutical companies signed a rare joint pledge promising not to seek regulatory approval before the safety and efficacy of their experimental vaccines are established in Phase 3 clinical trials. Dr. Anthony Fauci said experts would most likely know whether a vaccine is safe and effective by the end of 2020. Fauci added that it's *"unlikely"* a vaccine would be ready before the election.

President Trump is considering an "emergency use authorization" for a Covid-19 vaccine before Phase 3 clinical trials are completed. The CDC has instructed the states to be ready to distribute a vaccine by November 1. Rushing out a vaccine before it has been vetted as safe and effective is a risky gamble (31). An early 1976 outbreak of a new strain of the H1N1 swine flu virus at Fort Dix prompted the Ford administration to fast track a vaccine to prevent an epidemic. The vaccine was released in the fall and 45 million Americans were vaccinated. Side effects: 450 developed Guillain-Barre syndrome; more than 30 died. The vaccination program was cancelled. The swine flu claimed the life of only one soldier.

Finally, everything that I have learned about Covid-19 just reinforces what we've heard from the experts: it's contagious, insidious and potentially lethal. So, in the words of the late Hill Street Blues icon Michael Conrad, until a safe, effective vaccine is developed, and a significant percentage of the most vulnerable Americans have received it, *"Let's be careful out there!"*

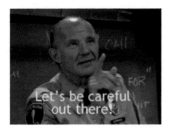

References

1. The COVID-19 Pandemic – How is the U.S. doing? by John Dalton, FHFMA, Garden State Focus, Spring 2020, Vol. 66, Num 2

2. Coronavirus: Why Spain is seeing second wave, by *James Badcock*, BBC News, 8/20/20

3. A pandemic lesson from Chile: Data transparency can save lives, by Khalida Sawari, News from Northeastern, 8/17/20

4. Coronavirus: Did 'herd immunity' change the course of the outbreak?, by Noel Titheradge and Dr Faye Kirkland, BBC News, 7/20/20

5. When Covid-19 Hit, Many Elderly Were Left to Die, by Matina Stevis-Gridneff, Matt Apuzzo and Monika Pronczuk, New York Times, 8/9/20

6. New Zealand has eliminated Coronavirus, Associated Press, 6/8/20

7. How South Korea Flattened the Curve, by Max Fisher and Choe Sang-Hun, 3/24/20

8. How Slovakia Flattened the Curve, by Miroslav Beblavy, FP Insider Access, 5/6/20

9. Identifying airborne transmission as the dominant route for the spread of COVID-19, by Renyi Zhang, Yixin Li, Annie L. Zhang, Yuan Wang and Mario J Molina. Proceedings of the National Academy of Sciences, 6/11/20

10. Community Use of Face Masks and Covid-19, by Wei Lyu and George L. Wehby, Health Affairs, 6/16/20

11. Smell dysfunction: a biomarker for COVID-19, by Shima T. Moein MD, Phd, Seyed Mohammad Reza Hashemian, MD, FCCM, Babak Mansourafshar, MD and others, International Forum of Allergy & Rhinology, 4/14/20

12. The odd, growing list of COVID-19 symptoms, explained, by Umair Irfan and Brian Resnick, Vox, 7/29/20

13. Clues to Why Covid-19 Hits Men Harder Than Women, by Robert Preidt, HealthDay News, 8/28/20

14. What Do Coronavirus Racial Disparities Look Like State by State? By Maria Gogoy, Daniel Wood, NPR, 5/30/20

15. Doctors studying why obesity may be tied to serious Covid-19, Associated Press, 9/9/20

16. If I Hadn't Been Transferred, I Would Have Died, by Daniela J. Lamas, New York Times, 8/4/20

17. Why Surviving Covid Might Come Down to Which NYC Hospital Admits You, by Brian M. Rosenthal, Joseph Goldstein, Sharon Otterman and Sheri Fink, The New York Times, 7/1/20

18. COVID-19 long-term toll signals billions in healthcare costs ahead, by Caroline Humer, Nick Brown; Emilio Parodi and Alistair Smout; Reuters, 8/3/20

19. Long-term symptoms, complications of Covid-19, by DeeDee Stiepan, Mayo Health Clinic News, 8/3/20

20. Mount Sinai, Yale, Johns Hopkins to track chronic kidney disease in Covid survivors, by John Gilmore, Modern Healthcare, 8/11/20

21. Covid-19 'long haulers' have lingering health problems, by Jay Greene, Crain's Detroit Business, 8/16/20

22. A Supercomputer Analyzed Covid-19 – and an Interesting New Theory Has Emerged, by Thomas Smith, Elemental, 9/1/20

23. A German Exception? Why the Country's Death Rate Is Low by Katrin Bennhold, New York Times, 4/4/20

24. Lessons Learned from Lombardy, Associated Press, 4/26/20

25. We should have done more, admits architect of Sweden's Covid-19 strategy, by Jon Henley, The Guardian, 6/3/20

26. Measuring the Covid-19 Policy Response Around the World, by Avik Roy, Foundation for Research on Equal Opportunity, 6/23/20

27. What the Pandemic Reveals About the Male Ego, by Nicholas Kristof, New York Times, 6/13/20

28. Coronavirus: Things the US has got wrong – and got right, by Anthony Zurcher, North America reporter, BBC News, 4/1/20

29. Operation Warp Speed promised to do the impossible. How far has it come? by Helen Branswell, Matthew Herper, Lev Facher, Ed Silverman ad Nicholas Florko, STAT, 9/8/20

30. Don't expect a coronavirus vaccine before the election — here's the likely timeline according to doctors, government officials, and analysts, by Aria Bendix, Business Insider, 9/9/20

31. Gerald Ford Rushed Out a Vaccine. It was a Fiasco, by Rick Perlstein, The New York Times, 9/2/2020

*　*　*　*　*　*

Table 1. Confirmed Cases and Fatality Rates, OECD Countries as of 9/20/2020

Confirmed Cases (1)	Fatalities (1)	Fatality Rate (%)	37 OECD Countries	Population (2)	Cases per 100,000	Fatalities per 100,000
1,815	25	1.4%	New Zealand	4,886,000	37.1	0.51
6,677	39	0.6%	Slovak Republic	5,450,000	122.5	0.72
22,975	383	1.7%	South Korea	51,640,000	44.5	0.74
79,142	1,508	1.9%	Japan	127,298,000	62.2	1.18
1,525	36	2.4%	Latvia	1,920,000	79.4	1.88
2,307	10	0.4%	Iceland	350,374	658.4	2.85
3,744	87	2.3%	Lithuania	2,794,329	134.0	3.11
14,978	338	2.3%	Greece	10,720,000	139.7	3.15
26,898	849	3.2%	Australia	24,990,000	107.6	3.40
48,306	502	1.0%	Czech Republic	10,650,000	453.6	4.71
2,924	64	2.2%	Estonia	1,329,000	220.0	4.82
12,883	266	2.1%	Norway	5,368,000	240.0	4.96
79,240	2,293	2.9%	Poland	37,970,000	208.7	6.04
8,980	339	3.8%	Finland	5,570,000	161.2	6.09
4,420	134	3.0%	Slovenia	2,081,000	212.4	6.44
17,990	683	3.8%	Hungary	9,773,000	184.1	6.99
38,095	766	2.0%	Austria	8,859,000	430.0	8.65
301,348	7,506	2.5%	Turkey	82,000,000	367.5	9.15
23,550	638	2.7%	Denmark	5,806,000	405.6	10.99
273,965	9,390	3.4%	Germany	83,020,000	330.0	11.31
183,602	1,236	0.7%	Israel	8,884,000	2,066.7	13.91
68,577	1,912	2.8%	Portugal	10,280,000	667.1	18.60
7,718	124	1.6%	Luxembourg	613,894	1,257.2	20.20
49,283	2,045	4.1%	Switzerland	8,570,000	575.1	23.86
144,699	9,267	6.4%	Canada	37,600,000	384.8	24.65
32,593	1,792	5.5%	Ireland	4,904,000	664.6	36.54
98,105	6,324	6.4%	Netherlands	17,280,000	567.7	36.60
467,614	31,257	6.7%	France	66,990,000	698.0	46.66
758,398	24,039	3.2%	Colombia	49,650,000	1,527.5	48.42
694,121	73,258	10.6%	Mexico	128,600,000	539.8	56.97
88,237	5,865	6.6%	Sweden	10,230,000	862.5	57.33
298,156	35,707	12.0%	Italy	60,360,000	494.0	59.16
6,769,370	199,411	2.9%	United States	327,700,000	2,065.7	60.85
392,845	41,866	10.7%	United Kingdom	66,270,000	592.8	63.17
640,040	30,495	4.8%	Spain	46,940,000	1,363.5	64.97
446,274	12,286	2.8%	Chile	18,730,000	2,382.7	65.60
100,748	9,944	9.9%	Belgium	11,460,000	879.1	86.77
12,212,142	512,684	4.2%	Total OECD	1,357,536,597	899.6	37.8

DATA SOURCES: 1. Johns Hopkins Coronavirus Resource Center. 2. Organisation for Economic Co-operation and Development, World Bank

The COVID-19 Pandemic – How is the U.S. doing? Part 3

By John J. Dalton, FHFMA

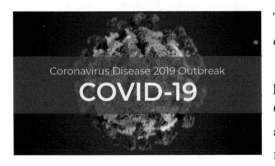

THE SHORT ANSWER – still not well, and with some added company.

Part 1, written May 1st for the Spring issue, compared America's pandemic performance with the other member countries of the Organisation for Economic Co-operation and Development (OECD) as of April 30 (1). With 61,931 deaths and a fatality rate of 19.4/100,000 residents, the U.S. ranked 29th among the 37 OECD members.

By Part 2, written September 21st for the Fall issue, the U.S. had slipped to 33rd place in the OECD, trailed only by Spain, Chile, the United Kingdom (UK) and Belgium (2). November 30 finds the U.S. in a virtual dead heat with Mexico and Chile for 31st place, then trailed by the UK, Italy, Spain and Belgium (see Chart 1: Covid-19 Fatality Rates, 20 OECD Members, 11/30/20). Table 1 - Confirmed Cases and Fatality Rates, OECD Countries as of 11/30/2020 displays the underlying data. With more than 270,000 deaths and a fatality rate of 81.66/100,00, COVID-19 has wiped out the equivalent of the entire population of the author's Jersey City hometown.

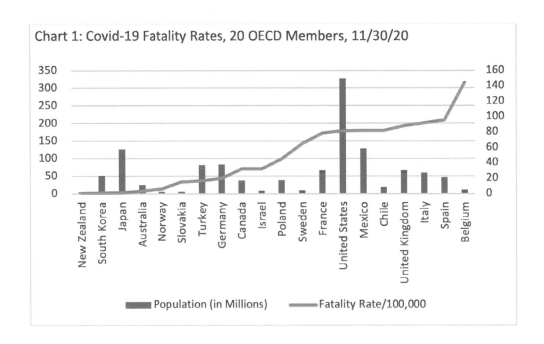

New Zealand, South Korea, Japan and Australia continue to lead the OECD in controlling the coronavirus. Their successful approaches were described in Part 1 of this series. Within the U.S., states with the highest fatality rates continue to be those hit early (Louisiana, Connecticut, Massachusetts, New York and New Jersey), but others have begun to close the gap after the Sunbelt's summer surge (see Chart 2: Covid-19 Fatality Rates, 20 Selected States, 11/30/20). More recently, the Mountain and Plains states are experiencing an overwhelming surge following the annual Sturgis Motorcycle Rally (3). That super spreader event drew nearly 500,000 to the small South Dakota town from August 7-16. Kaiser Family Foundation epidemiologist Josh Michaud said: "*Holding a half-million-person rally in the midst of a pandemic is emblematic of a nation as a whole that maybe isn't taking [the novel coronavirus] as seriously as we should.*"

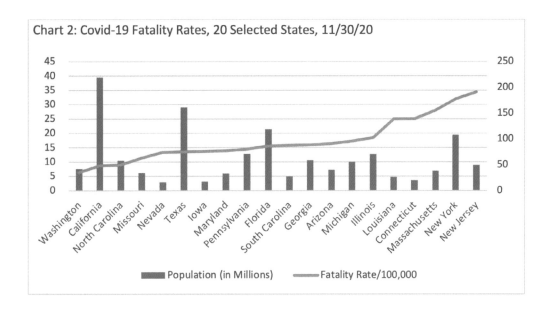

Second Surge in Central Europe

THE ELEVEN WEEKS FROM September 20 through November 30 witnessed the rapid rise of COVID-19's second surge, striking ten OECD members in Central Europe with a vengeance (see Chart 3: Fatality Rates, Central Europe, 9/20-11/30/20). Previously, Slovakia had the lowest fatality rate in the Western Hemisphere at 0.72/100,000 thanks to a March 16 national lockdown with universal compliance. Its fatality rate increased twentyfold to 14.67/100,000 by November 30. Likewise, the neighboring Czech Republic (Bohemia) experienced a fifteenfold increase from 4.71 to 77.68/100,000. Even Germany, which has maintained the lowest fatality rate among major Western democracies and canceled Oktoberfest, had a 75 percent increase in its fatality rate/100,000 from 11.81 to 19.85.

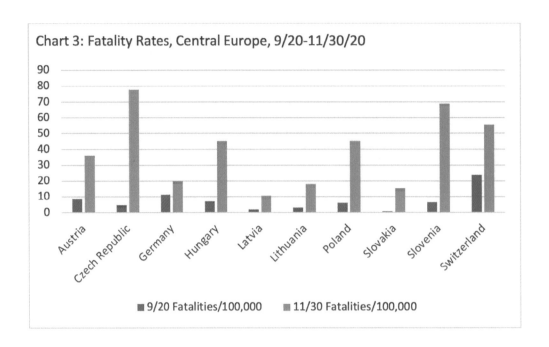

Chart 3: Fatality Rates, Central Europe, 9/20-11/30/20

■ 9/20 Fatalities/100,000   ■ 11/30 Fatalities/100,000

Clearly, COVID fatigue is both real and dangerous!

With more than 4 million confirmed cases during November, the U.S. is just weeks behind Central Europe's second surge as the country heads into a challenging winter. Dr. Robert Redfield, head of the CDC, warns that the pandemic will pose the country's grimmest public health crisis yet over the next few months, noting that the University of Washington's Institute for Health Metrics and Evaluation has projected the death toll could reach nearly 450,000 by March 1 (4). To place that amount in perspective, 415,399 American lives were lost during the 45 months of World War 2.

One of America's founding fathers, Thomas Paine said, *"These are the time that try men's souls."* (5) However, there is a light at the end of the tunnel: three vaccines have completed Phase 3 clinical trials with a high degree of effectiveness, and two already have applied to the FDA for emergency use authorization.

The Light at the End of the Tunnel

ON NOVEMBER 9, PFIZER and its partner, German drug maker BioNTechSE, announced that its COVID-19 vaccine may be 90% effective based on data from its phase 3 clinical trials (6). This interim analysis, from an independent data monitoring board, looked at 94 infections recorded so far in a study that has enrolled nearly 44,000 people in the U.S. and five other countries. For the vaccine to be 90% effective, nearly all the infections must have occurred in placebo recipients. The Pfizer vaccine consists of genetic material called mRNA encased in tiny particles that shuttle it into our cells, then trains the immune system to recognize the spiked protein on the surface of the virus. Since it's not made with the coronavirus itself, there's no chance anyone could catch it from the shots.

One week later, Moderna announced that its experimental vaccine was 94.5% effective in preventing disease, according to an analysis of its clinical trial (7). The Moderna study included 30,000 volunteers: half got two doses of the vaccine 28 days apart; half got two shots of a placebo on the same schedule. Of 95 instances of COVID-19 illness among the study participants, only five cases were in the vaccinated group. The Moderna vaccine also is based on mRNA, or messenger RNA.

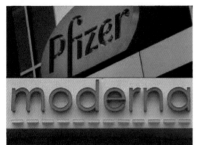

The Moderna and Pfizer studies were conducted using slightly different protocols. To be counted as a COVID-19 case, participants in the Moderna study had to have at least two symptoms of disease in addition to a positive test for the virus. The Pfizer study required only one symptom. Also, Moderna waited 14 days following the second injection to begin counting cases; Pfizer's study started counting at seven days.

Pharmaceutical giant Pfizer's chief executive, Dr. Albert Bourla, had chosen from the start to keep Pfizer at arm's length from the government's crash effort, Operation Warp Speed, and declined federal research and development money (8). Moderna, a much smaller biotech firm with 800 employees, received nearly $2.5 billion, teaming up with the National Institutes of Health's Vaccine Research Center on the scientific work in a successful partnership to develop, manufacture and sell its vaccine to the federal government. In a contest between David (Moderna) and Goliath (Pfizer), America won!

The encouraging late-stage trial results from Pfizer and Moderna have set a high bar for rival vaccines soon to follow (9). Both use messenger RNA technology that instructs cells to make copies of the coronavirus spike protein stimulating the creation of protective antibodies. Pfizer's vaccine requires deep freeze storage (-94F) but can be kept at refrigerator temperatures for as much as five days. Moderna's vaccine can be safely stored in freezers at about 25F and is stable at refrigerator temperatures for 30 days, which should ease distribution. Both companies are seeking emergency-use authorization from the U.S. Food and Drug Administration with Pfizer's review scheduled for December 10 and Moderna's review one week later. It's unclear how long protection will last or how many will refuse to be vaccinated. Ramping up production and distributing the doses also pose challenges.

On 11/23, Astra-Zeneca announced that its vaccine developed in the UK with Oxford University can protect 70.4% of people from becoming ill and up to 90% if a lower first dose is used (10). Chief Investigator Andrew Pollard, director of the Oxford Vaccine Group said, *"We think that by giving a smaller first dose that we're priming the immune system differently – we're setting it up better to respond."* The Astra-Zeneca vaccine uses a different technology than mRNA (it's a replication-deficient viral vector vaccine), is much less expensive, and requires only refrigerator storage (11). The UK has preordered 100 million doses. Novovax, Johnson & Johnson and several others also have various COVID-19 vaccines in phase 3 clinical trials.

The development of three promising vaccines in so short a period is an incredible achievement. Production and distribution challenges remain, but this is an important first step.

Vaccine Rollout Plans

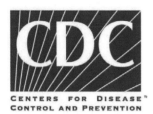

EXPERTS HAVE COMPARED THE logistical challenges of delivering vaccinations to hundreds of millions of Americans to the enormous efforts involved in gearing up industrial production during World War 2. Who should the vaccine be given to first? How will it be distributed and stored? Who will be allowed to administer injections? What records will be kept? All burning issues currently being addressed.

On December 1, The CDC's Advisory Committee on Immunization Practices (ACIP) voted 13 to 1 to put health care providers (21 million) and long-term care residents (3 million) at the top of the vaccine priority list (12). The ACIP has been meeting at least monthly since the spring, using mathematical models and ethical frameworks to try to determine how to best use scarce supplies of vaccine when the national vaccination effort begins. Next up are likely to be roughly 85 million "essential workers," followed by everyone over 65 and adults with medical conditions that put them at high risk of coronavirus infection, such as diabetes or obesity. However, state officials will also be responsible for ultimately deciding which residents are the first to get the vaccines.

A division of the Department of Homeland Security has compiled a list of essential workers that includes teachers and others who work in schools, emergency responders, police officers, grocery workers, corrections officers, public transit workers and others whose jobs make it hard or impossible to work from home. Pfizer and Moderna estimate that they will have enough to vaccinate 22.5 million Americans with the required two doses by year's end.

Moncef Slaoui, Operation Warp Speed's chief advisor, predicted that 100 million Americans would be immunized by the end of February (13). Outlining an ambitious timeline, Slaoui expects 20 million Americans to be vaccinated by year end, followed by 30 million in January and another 50 million in February. By then, "*we will have potentially immunized 100 million people, which is really more or less the size of the significant at-risk population: the elderly, the healthcare workers, the first-line workers, people with comorbidities,*" Slaoui said.

A recent research study conducted by Yale and Harvard examined vaccine efficacy and found that found that factors related to implementation will contribute more to the success of vaccination programs than a vaccine's efficacy as determined in clinical trials (14). They learned that the benefits of a vaccine will decline if manufacturing or deployment delays, significant concerns in the public about getting vaccinated or greater epidemic severity develops. They found that there is an urgent need for health officials to continue and expand efforts to promote public confidence in COVID-19 vaccines, and to encourage continued adherence to other mitigation approaches, even after a vaccine becomes available.

When interviewed by the New York Times about the study, Dr. A. David Paltiel, professor at the Yale School of Public Health, said "*Vaccines don't save lives. Vaccination programs save lives.*" (15) His study team concluded that to reduce the pandemic's infections, hospitalizations and deaths, a successful vaccine rollout was just as important as the vaccine's efficacy. Dr. Paltiel is concerned that the U.S. has not done enough to prepare for successful distribution of the vaccine in the months to come. This study makes it clear that mitigation measures along with a successful rollout of approved vaccines and public commitment to getting vaccinated are all important to controlling COVID-19.

Opposition is expected from COVID deniers and anti-vaxxers. However, if the rollout is successful, experts expect that the U.S. could return to a new normal by late April/early May by which time millions of the general public will have been vaccinated. The new normal likely will be quite different - social distancing and mask wearing in public are likely to be universal.

References

1. The COVID-19 Pandemic – How is the U.S. doing? by John Dalton, FHFMA, Garden State Focus, Spring 2020, Vol. 66, Num 2

2. The COVID-19 Pandemic – How is the U.S. doing? Part 2 by John Dalton, FHFMA, Garden State Focus, Fall 2020, Vol. 66, Num 3

3. How the Sturgis Motorcycle Rally may have spread the coronavirus across the Upper Midwest, by Brittany Shammas and Lena H. Sun, Washington Post, 10/17/20

4. CDC chief warns Americans face 'rough' winter from COVID-19 surge, by Steve Gorman, Daniel Trotta, Reuters, 12/2/20

5. The American Crisis, by Thomas Paine, December 1776

6. Pfizer says COVID-19 vaccine is looking 90% effective, by Lauran Nergaard and Linda A. Johnson, Associated Press, 11/10/20

7. Moderna's COVID-19 Vaccine Shines In Clinical Trial, by Joe Palca, NPR, 11/16/20

8. Politics, Science and the Remarkable Race for a Coronavirus Vaccine, New York Times, by Sharon LaFraniere, Katie Thomas, Noah Welland, David Gelles, Sheryl Gay Stolberg and Denise Grady, 11/21/20

9. Moderna, Pfizer Shots Look Strong: Here's How They Stack Up, by James Paton, Bloomberg 11/16/20

10. Oxford AstraZeneca Covid vaccine has up to 90% efficacy, data reveals, by Sarah Bosely and Ian Sample, The Guardian, 1/23/20

11. COVID-19 Vaccine Tracker, posted by Jeff Craven, Regulatory Affairs Professional Society, 12/3/20

12. Long-Term-Care Residents and Health Workers Should Get Vaccine First, C.D.C. Panel Says, by Amy Goodnough, New York Times, 12/1/20

13. Operation Warp Speed's top scientist predicts more than 100 million Americans could be immunized with coronavirus vaccines within the next 100 days, by Andrew Dunn, Business Insider, 12/2/20

14. Clinical Outcomes of a COVID-19 Vaccine: Implementation over Efficacy, by A. David Paltiel, Jason L. Schwartz, Amy Zheng and Rochelle P. Walensky, Health Affairs 11/19/20

15. 2 Companies Say Their Vaccines Are 95% Effective. What Does That Mean?, by Carl Zimmer, New York Times, 11/20/20

* * * * * *

Table 1. Confirmed Cases and Fatality Rates, OECD Countries as of 11/30/2020

Confirmed Cases (1)	Fatalities (1)	Fatality Rate (%)	37 OECD Countries	Population (2)	Cases per 100,000	Fatalities per 100,000
2,056	25	1.2%	New Zealand	4,886,000	42.1	0.51
34,201	526	1.5%	South Korea	51,640,000	66.2	1.02
148,945	2,075	1.4%	Japan	127,298,000	117.0	1.63
27,904	908	3.3%	Australia	24,990,000	111.7	3.63
35,971	332	0.9%	Norway	5,368,000	670.1	6.18
24,912	399	1.6%	Finland	5,570,000	447.3	7.16
5,392	26	0.5%	Iceland	350,374	1,538.9	7.42
12,308	118	1.0%	Estonia	1,329,000	926.1	8.88
17,075	206	1.2%	Latvia	1,920,000	889.3	10.73
81,002	837	1.0%	Denmark	5,806,000	1,395.1	14.42
105,929	839	0.8%	Slovak Republic	5,450,000	1,943.7	15.39
638,487	13,746	2.2%	Turkey	82,000,000	778.6	16.76
61,325	506	0.8%	Lithuania	2,794,329	2,194.6	18.11
1,069,491	16,480	1.5%	Germany	83,020,000	1,288.2	19.85
105,271	2,406	2.3%	Greece	10,720,000	982.0	22.44
377,499	12,093	3.2%	Canada	37,600,000	1,004.0	32.16
336,160	2,864	0.9%	Israel	8,884,000	3,783.9	32.24
282,456	3,184	1.1%	Austria	8,859,000	3,188.4	35.94
72,544	2,053	2.8%	Ireland	4,904,000	1,479.3	41.86
298,061	4,505	1.5%	Portugal	10,280,000	2,899.4	43.82
990,811	17,150	1.7%	Poland	37,970,000	2,609.5	45.17
217,122	4,823	2.2%	Hungary	9,773,000	2,221.7	49.35
34,678	321	0.9%	Luxembourg	613,894	5,648.9	52.29
531,911	9,453	1.8%	Netherlands	17,280,000	3,078.2	54.70
327,072	4,753	1.5%	Switzerland	8,570,000	3,816.5	55.46
243,129	6,681	2.7%	Sweden	10,230,000	2,376.6	65.31
75,806	1,435	1.9%	Slovenia	2,081,000	3,642.8	68.96
1,308,376	36,584	2.8%	Colombia	49,650,000	2,635.2	73.68
521,132	8,273	1.6%	Czech Republic	10,650,000	4,893.3	77.68
2,274,579	52,816	2.3%	France	66,990,000	3,395.4	78.84
13,492,101	**267,600**	**2.0%**	**United States**	**327,700,000**	**4,117.2**	**81.66**
1,107,071	105,655	9.5%	Mexico	128,600,000	860.9	82.16
551,743	15,410	2.8%	Chile	18,730,000	2,945.8	82.27
1,633,652	58,545	3.6%	United Kingdom	66,270,000	2,465.1	88.34
1,601,554	55,576	3.5%	Italy	60,360,000	2,653.3	92.07
1,648,187	45,069	2.7%	Spain	46,940,000	3,511.3	96.01
576,599	16,547	2.9%	Belgium	11,460,000	5,031.4	144.39
30,872,512	770,819	2.5%	Total OECD	1,357,536,597	2,274.2	56.8

DATA SOURCES: 1. Johns Hopkins Coronavirus Resource Center. 2. Organisation for Economic Co-operation and Development, World Bank

The COVID-19 Pandemic – How is the U.S. doing? Part 4

By John J. Dalton, FHFMA

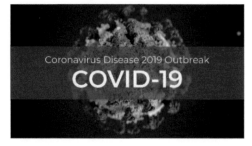

THE SHORT ANSWER – the roller coaster ride continues with vaccines vs. virus variants in the race to recovery. The key issue facing the U.S. is whether a Spring Break/Passover/Easter surge can be avoided, unlike the Thanksgiving/Hanukah/Christmas surge that led to more than 95,000 deaths in January. More on that later, but first, some brief background.

On December 31, 2019, the government in Wuhan, China, confirmed that health authorities were treating dozens of cases of a pneumonia of unknown origin. Three weeks later, the United States confirmed its first case in Washington state – a man in his 30s developed symptoms after returning from Wuhan. The World Health Organization (WHO) declared a global health emergency on January 30 and subsequently named the disease Covid-19, an acronym for coronavirus disease 2019. On March 11, the WHO declared Covid-19 a global pandemic.

Meanwhile, during February, more than 2.2 million travelers arrived in New York from Europe, some already infected by the novel coronavirus. New Jersey's first case was confirmed March 5. Shortly thereafter, the New York Metro Area joined Milan and Madrid as the global epicenters of the worst pandemic in over a century, and the author began tracking and reporting on the performance of the 37 member nations of the Organisation for Economic Co-operation and Development (OECD) in dealing with the pandemic. The key metric tracked is fatality rate per 100,000 residents.

The first three parts of this series were written May 1, September 21 and November 30, 2020, respectively. This 4th (and hopefully final) article is written as of March 31, 2021, a full year after the WHO's global pandemic declaration. Over the course of the past year, Australia, Japan, New Zealand and South Korea have consistently led the OECD in protecting their residents from Covid-19. On the other hand, Belgium, Italy, the U.K. and the U.S. have consistently ranked in the bottom quartile of the OECD with the highest fatality rates in the developed world.

Biden Declares War on Pandemic

INAUGURATED THE DAY AFTER America's death toll surpassed 400,000, President Joe Biden wasted no time attacking the pandemic (1). That afternoon, his first three Executive Orders targeted Covid-19: requiring masks on federal property, rejoining the World Health Organization and establishing a White House Covid-19 response team led by Jeff Zients. Biden's executive actions were also intended to set an example for state and local officials as they try to rein in the virus and drew praise from U.S. Chamber of Commerce President Suzanne Clark calling it "*a smart and practical approach.*"

The series of Executive orders and presidential directives issued during President Biden's first full day in office signaled a more centralized federal response to the spread of Covid-19, including:(2)

- Ramping up the pace of manufacturing and testing.

- Requiring mask wearing during interstate travel.

- Establishing a Pandemic Testing Board.

- Establishing a health equity task force.

- Publishing guidance for schools and workers.

- Finding more treatments for Covid-19 and future pandemics.

Agencies also were directed to identify areas where the administration could invoke the Defense Production Act to increase manufacturing, such as PPE, swabs, reagents, pipettes and syringes. The orders Biden signed were aimed at jump starting his national Covid-19 strategy to increase vaccinations and testing, lay the groundwork for reopening schools and businesses, and immediately increase the use of masks. Promising stringent adherence to public health guidance, Biden declared: *"To a nation waiting for action, let me be clear on this point: help is on the way."*(3)

Is the strategy working? Let's look at where America stands at day 70 of the Biden Administration.

#30 of 37 in the OECD

WITH 551,747 COVID-19 DEATHS as of March 31, the U.S. fatality rate of 166.7/100,000 ranked 30th of the 37 OECD member nations, just below Portugal in the bottom quartile (see Table 1: Confirmed Cases and Fatality Rates, OECD Countries as of 3/31/2021). The U.S. is trailed by Slovakia, Italy, the U.K., Slovenia, Belgium, Hungary and the Czech Republic. Part 3 of this series highlighted the alarming increase in fatality rates in Central Europe that began in the Fall.

Chart 1.

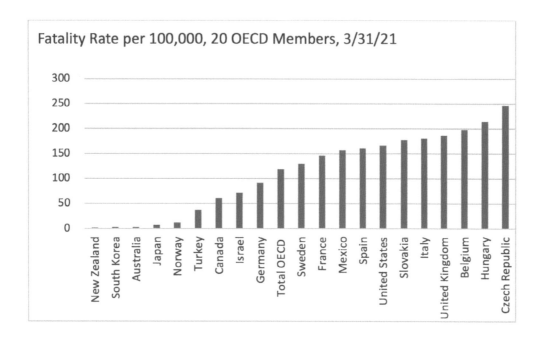

Fatality Rate per 100,000, 20 OECD Members, 3/31/21

Covid-19 has continued to rage, and Hungary and the Czech Republic have displaced Belgium with the highest fatality rates among OECD member nations (see Chart 1: "Fatality Rate per 100,000, 20 OECD Members, 3/31/21"). Nonetheless, Hungary's Prime Minister Viktor Orban has said that his government will not tighten restrictions and is determined to continue moving to reopen society (4). After a month of lockdown measures to combat the virus, Mr. Orban said, the plan to reopen stores after Easter, followed by schools and then restaurants and hotels, would not change.

Conversely, New Zealand, Australia, South Korea, Japan and four of the Scandanavian countries (Norway, Finland, Iceland and Denmark) continue to rank in the first quartile, just ahead of Canada at #10. Sweden remains the outlier among the Scandanavian countries at #23 with a fatality rate of 129.8/100,000. Sweden's flawed attempt at herd immunity had it at #33 of 37 as late as July 30, 2020.

Last week, on a CNN documentary titled "COVID WAR: The Pandemic Doctors Speak Out,"(5) Dr. Deborah Birx, a member of Trump's White House coronavirus response team, said that although the first 100,000 deaths were unavoidable, *"the rest of them, in my mind, could have been mitigated or decreased substantially."* Birx added: *"The majority of the people in the White House did not take this seriously."* Brett Giroir, the nation's coronavirus testing chief under Trump, admitted, *"When we said there were millions of tests available, there weren't.... There were components of the test available, but not the full... deal."* Former director of the CDC Robert Redfield said that Health and Human Services Secretary Alex Azar personally tried to change scientific reports that the White House didn't like. Former HHS Secretary Azar denies Redfield's assertion.

Whatever the ultimate truth, it's clear that the Trump Administration's failure to take the pandemic seriously resulted in well over 100,000 avoidable American deaths:

- If the U.S. had merely matched the OECD's average fatality rate/100,000 of 119.3, 157,000 more Americans would be alive today.
- If the U.S. had matched Germany's performance, 250,000 more Americans would be alive today.
- If the U.S. had matched the Scandanavian countries, 339,000 more Americans would be alive today.
- If the U.S. had matched Canada, 350,000 more Americans would be alive today.

Turning to the data from the states, the fatality rates for the Northeastern states that were the global epicenter of the pandemic last March and April continue to rank among the highest in the developed world (see Chart 2: "Fatality Rate/100,000, Selected States, 3/31/21"). To place the state data in perspective, the Czech Republic's fatality rate of 246.7/100,000 is the highest in the OECD, tied with Massachusetts, but lower than either New York or New Jersey.

As noted earlier, America's first confirmed case of Covid-19 occurred in Washington state, followed by an outbreak in a Kirkland nursing home. The state reacted immediately and has continued to protect its residents better than the OECD's average (see Table 2: Ten states change in fatality rates, 9 months ended 3/31/21). Washington's fatality rate of 68.7/100,000 would place it in at #12 in the OECD, between Estonia and Israel. Despite a winter surge in Southern California that had ICUs running out of capacity, the state's fatality rate of 142.2/100,000 remains below the U.S. average of 154.8/100,000 and equivalent to #25 in the OECD, between Lithuania and France.

Chart 2.

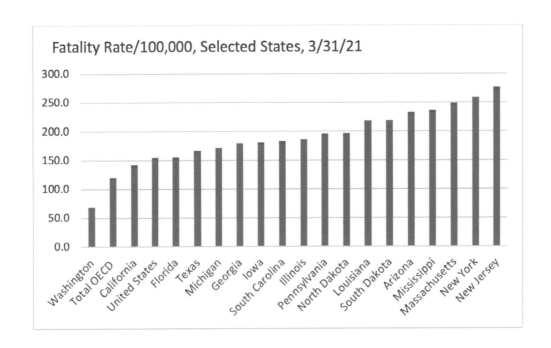

After being overwhelmed from mid-March through April 2020, New York and New Jersey's fatality rates have been below the U.S. average of 116.2/100,000 for the nine months ended March 31, 2021. Massachusetts and Pennsylvania have been less successful in controlling the pandemic, as have several of the Sunbelt states (e.g., Arizona, Georgia, Florida, South Carolina and Texas). And, as reported in Part 3, the annual Sturgis, South Dakota Motorcycle Rally from August 7-16 was a super spreader event on steroids, producing surges throughout the North Central Midwest and Mountain states.

Table 2. Ten states change in fatality rates, 9 months ended 3/31/21

State	06/30/20	03/31/21	Difference	% Change
Washington	17.3	68.7	51.4	297.1%
OECD Average	**26.2**	**119.3**	**93.1**	**355.3%**
New York	161.5	258.6	97.1	60.1%
New Jersey	169.1	276.3	107.2	63.4%
Michigan	62.0	171.4	109.4	176.5%
United States	**38.6**	**154.8**	**116.2**	**301.0%**
California	15.2	142.2	127.0	835.5%
Massachusetts	117.3	248.5	131.2	111.8%
Florida	16.3	155.6	139.3	853.4%
Pennsylvania	51.9	195.9	144.0	277.5%
Georgia	26.4	179.4	153.0	579.5%
Texas	8.3	166.4	158.1	1904.8%

Vaccine Rollout

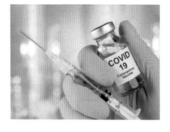

ON DECEMBER 8, PRESIDENT-ELECT Biden set a goal of administering 100 million vaccine doses in his first 100 days (6). That goal was reached on day 58, and the U.S. now is on pace to administer more than 200 million doses in the first 100 days. On March 11, the one-year anniversary of the WHO's global pandemic declaration, President Biden urged all states, tribes and territories to make all American adults eligible for a Covid-19 vaccine by May 1 (7).

On February 27, the Food and Drug Administration issued an emergency use authorization (EUA) for Johnson & Johnson's adenovirus vaccine, further expanding the availability of safe effective vaccines for Covid-19 (8). The vaccine was 72% effective in the US, compared to 66% in Latin America and 57% in South Africa. Unlike the Pfizer/BioNTech and Moderna mRNA-based vaccines, J&J's Janssen vaccine requires only one injection and can be stored for at least three months at 36-46F. Novavax expects data from a 30,000-person trial in the United States and Mexico by early April. A late-stage trial in the UK found Novavax's vaccine 96% effective against Covid-19's original variant and 86% effective in protecting against the more contagious B.1.1.7 variant (9).

With Americans being vaccinated at a rate of 3 million per day, more than 154 million doses have been administered. Nearly 100 million have received at least one shot and 56.1 million are fully vaccinated, 17.1% of the U.S. population.

The wild card in the equation is the emergence of virulent variants as the novel coronavirus continues to mutate. Of particular concern are the Brazilian, British and South African variants, all of which are more highly transmissible. However, all three vaccines with FDA approval have proven effective in preventing severe disease against the variants.

With ample vaccine supplies, the U.S. now is in a vaccine vs. virus variants race to recovery, providing that a Spring Break/Passover/Easter surge can be avoided, unlike the Thanksgiving/Hanukah/Christmas surge that led to 95,000 deaths in January.

The American Rescue Plan Act

THE MARCH 11 ENACTMENT of the $1.9 trillion American Rescue Plan Act (ARPA) contains the most extensive health insurance improvements for Americans since the Affordable Care Act (ACA) became law 11 years ago (10). The law temporarily extends the eligibility criteria for ACA subsidies to include people with incomes above 400% of the federal poverty level so that no one must pay more than 8.5% of their income on insurance premiums. The Congressional Budget Office estimates that the ACA changes will extend coverage to 2.5 million uninsured Americans. The federal government will cover 100% of COBRA premiums for laid-off workers between April 1 and September 30. The package also offers two years of additional federal funding to encourage Medicaid expansion in the 12 states that have not extended coverage to low-income adults.

The ARPA also contains important provisions to deal with the economic consequences of the pandemic, including $1,400 stimulus checks, expansion of the child tax credit, support for low-income families and child-care facilities, and rent support. Economists estimate that the poorest fifth of Americans will experience a more than 20 percent increase in their incomes. The ARPA should reduce poverty by one-third, reducing the number of people living below the federal poverty level from 44 million to 28 million. While these provisions are not directed at healthcare, they improve the social determinants of health, the conditions in the places where people live, learn, work, and play that affect a wide range of health and quality-of life-risks and outcomes.

In a related development, President Biden extended a special enrollment period to allow people to sign up for health insurance through the federal health insurance marketplace through August 15 (11). The extended open enrollment period will allow Americans to take advantage of new savings under ARPA. However, the ARPA subsidy provisions are temporary, lasting for two years, retroactive to January 1, 2021.

A Return to Normal?

AFTER A YEAR OF riding the Covid-19 roller coaster, Americans yearn for nothing less than a return to a normal lifestyle. In a recent article in the Atlantic, Joe Pinsker lays out a timeline for a likely return to a new normal (12). He expects an uncertain spring, an amazing summer, a cautious fall and winter, and finally, relief.

Given that the wild card is the potential emergence of virulent vaccine-resistant variants, daily life will continue to be far from normal for the next few months. By late spring, small gatherings of vaccinated people should be feasible. At some point between June and September, the combination of widespread vaccinations and warmer weather may make many activities much safer, including taking public transit, being in a workplace, dining inside restaurants, and traveling domestically. However, experts don't foresee the return of indoor concerts, full stadiums or high levels of international travel yet.

The summer reprieve could be temporary. Some resurgence of the virus is likely in the fall as activities move indoors. If stubborn variants do circulate, new vaccines should be able to tame them relatively quickly. While there might be a need to revert to some of the precautions from earlier in the pandemic, the disruptions to daily life are likely to be short-lived. Beyond next winter, experts' predict a return to whatever qualifies as normal in the post-pandemic future. The virus will still exist, but like the flu it will circulate primarily in the colder months.

This author for one hopes that Mr. Pinsker is correct. Meanwhile, wash your hands, watch your distance and wear a mask.

References

1. Biden looks to galvanize Covid-19 fight, vaccinations as he takes office, by Susan Heavey, Patricia Zengerle, Reuters, 1/21/21

2. Here's What's in Biden's Executive Orders Aimed at Curbing the Pandemic, by Noah Weiland, New York Times, 1/22/21

3. Biden signs burst of virus orders, vows "Help is on the way", by Ricardo Alonso-Zakduvar and Zeke Miller, Associated Press, 1/21/21

4. Hungary, despite having one of the world's worst per capita death rates, plans to ease restrictions, by Benjamin Novak, New York Times, 4/1/21

5. COVID WAR: The Pandemic Doctors Speak Out, hosted by Dr. Sanjay Gupta, CNN, 3/28/21

6. Biden Promises 100 Million Vaccine Shots in 100 Days, but Shortage Worries Rise, by Sheryl Gay Stolberg and Sharon LaFranier, New York Times, 12/8/20

7. Biden directs states to make all adults eligible for COVID vaccines by May 1, by Joey Garrison, USA Today, 3/11/21

8. Johnson & Johnson Applies for Emergency Use Authorization for COVID-19 Vaccine, by Phil Galewitz, Kaiser Health News, 1/29/21

9. Novovax vaccine 96% effective against original coronavirus, 86% vs British variant in UK trial, by Dania Nadeem, Carl O'Donnell, Reuters, 3/11/21

10. Will the American Rescue Plan Act Reduce the Number of Uninsured Americans, by Sara R. Collins and Gabriella Aboulafia, The Commonwealth Fund, 3/22/21

11. Biden Extends Health Insurance Marketplace Through Summer, by Chelsea Cirruzzo, U.S. News & World Report, 3/23/21

12. The Most Likely Timeline for Life to Return to Normal, by Joe Pinsker, The Atlantic, 2/24/21

Table 1. Confirmed Cases and Fatality Rates, OECD Countries as of 3/31/2021

Rank	Confirmed Cases (1)	Fatalities (1)	Fatality Rate (%)	37 OECD Countries	Population (2)	Cases per 100,000	Fatalities per 100,000
1	2,497	26	1.0%	New Zealand	4,822,233	51.8	0.54
2	103,088	1,731	1.7%	South Korea	51,269,185	201.1	3.38
3	29,304	909	3.1%	Australia	25,499,884	114.9	3.56
4	474,566	9,155	1.9%	Japan	126,476,461	375.2	7.24
5	6,205	29	0.5%	Iceland	341,243	1,818.4	8.50
6	95,695	673	0.7%	Norway	5,421,241	1,765.2	12.41
7	77,452	844	1.1%	Finland	5,540,720	1,397.9	15.23
8	3,317,182	31,537	1.0%	Turkey	84,339,067	3,933.1	37.39
9	231,295	2,420	1.0%	Denmark	5,792,202	3,993.2	41.78
10	984,963	22,936	2.3%	Canada	37,742,154	2,609.7	60.77
11	106,424	902	0.8%	Estonia	1,326,535	8,022.7	68.00
12	833,040	6,203	0.7%	Israel	8,655,535	9,624.4	71.67
13	263,689	8,093	3.1%	Greece	10,423,054	2,529.9	77.65
14	2,828,870	76,459	2.7%	Germany	83,783,942	3,376.4	91.26
15	235,854	4,587	1.9%	Ireland	4,937,786	4,776.5	92.90
16	1,292,218	16,686	1.3%	Netherlands	17,134,872	7,541.5	97.38
17	102,363	1,899	1.9%	Latvia	1,886,198	5,426.9	100.68
18	546,229	9,339	1.7%	Austria	9,006,398	6,064.9	103.69
19	61,642	746	1.2%	Luxembourg	625,978	9,847.3	119.17
20	601,124	10,334	1.7%	Switzerland	8,654,622	6,945.7	119.40
21	995,538	23,135	2.3%	Chile	19,116,201	5,207.8	121.02
22	2,397,731	63,255	2.6%	Colombia	50,882,891	4,712.3	124.31
23	804,886	13,465	1.7%	Sweden	10,377,781	7,755.9	129.75
24	216,119	3,574	1.7%	Lithuania	2,722,289	7,938.9	131.29
25	4,646,127	95,502	2.1%	France	65,273,511	7,117.9	146.31
26	2,321,717	56,045	2.4%	Poland	37,846,611	6,134.5	148.08
27	2,232,910	202,633	9.1%	Mexico	128,932,753	1,731.8	157.16
28	3,284,353	75,459	2.3%	Spain	46,754,778	7,024.6	161.39
29	821,722	16,848	2.1%	Portugal	10,196,709	8,058.7	165.23
30	**30,467,755**	**551,747**	**1.8%**	**United States**	**331,002,561**	**9,204.7**	**166.69**
31	361,185	9,719	2.7%	Slovak Republic	5,459,642	6,615.5	178.02
32	3,584,899	109,346	3.1%	Italy	60,461,826	5,929.2	180.85
33	4,359,921	126,955	2.9%	United Kingdom	67,886,011	6,422.4	187.01
34	215,602	4,047	1.9%	Slovenia	2,078,938	10,370.8	194.67
35	876,842	22,966	2.6%	Belgium	11,589,623	7,565.8	198.16
36	652,433	20,737	3.2%	Hungary	9,660,351	6,753.7	214.66
37	1,532,232	26,421	1.7%	Czech Republic	10,708,981	14,307.9	246.72
	71,965,672	1,627,362	2.3%	Total OECD	1,364,630,767	5,273.6	119.3

DATA SOURCES: 1. Johns Hopkins Coronavirus Resource Center. 2. Organisation for Economic Co-operation and Development, World Bank

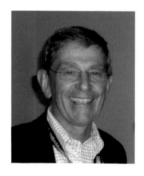

JOHN J. DALTON, FHFMA, IS SENIOR ADVISER EMERITUS AT BESLER AND CO-FOUNDER of the Healing American Healthcare Coalition where he serves as Editor of its twice-monthly newsletter, the Three Minute Read™. *A* Past President of the New Jersey Chapter of the Healthcare Financial Management Association, he served on the National Board from 1994-96 and received HFMA's Individual Lifetime Achievement Award in 2001.

In 50 years of healthcare involvement as consumer, consultant, employer, regulator and hospital trustee, John has authored dozens of articles on revenue cycle management, uncompensated care and healthcare policy issues. His 2016 three-part series in ***garden state focus***, *"American Healthcare: Worst Value in the Developed World?"* was cited in the first book in this series. A former Deloitte partner, John managed the design and implementation of New Jersey's first hospital rate setting system and helped design the country's first inpatient payment system based on diagnosis-related groups (DRGs). It became the basis for Medicare's Inpatient Prospective Payment System, still in use today.

John has served on the Boards of Children's Specialized Hospital, the Robert Wood Johnson Healthcare Corporation and St. Joseph's Health. The New Jersey Hospital Association named him as its 2017 Hospital Trustee of the Year. He earned a bachelor's degree in mechanical engineering from Stevens Institute of Technology where he received its 2013 Alumni Award and an MBA in Finance from Illinois Institute of Technology.

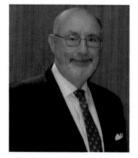

EDWARD C. EICHHORN IS president of the Medilink Consulting Group LLC and co-founder of the Healing American Healthcare Coalition. Ed is also co-author of *"Healing American Healthcare, A Plan to Provide Quality Care for All While Saving $1 Trillion a Year."* He has written commentary for US News & World Report, Smerconish.com, HR.com, Law 360, Managed Health Care Executive Magazine, and ***garden state focus***, among others.

Ed began his career more than 45 years ago as a medical device development engineer. During his career he has been the director of research and development for a kidney dialysis company. He helped to found and later sell an innovative mobile medical testing business. Ed has been a senior executive for a large chain of medical imaging centers with responsibility for sales, marketing, and strategic planning. At the Medilink Consulting Group Ed advises clients on marketing, strategic planning, and healthcare policy issues.

He earned a bachelor's degree in engineering from Stevens Institute of Technology and an MBA in Industrial Management from Fairleigh Dickinson University. Ed has a long-standing interest in serving his community. He served on his local school board for 12 years and on the board of trustees at his alma mater for 3 years.